STEM
CELL
REVOLUTION

STEM CELL CELL REVOLUTION

JOSEPH CHRISTIANO, ND, CNC, CNHP

SILOAM

Most CHARISMA HOUSE BOOK GROUP products are available at special quantity discounts for bulk purchase for sales promotions, premiums, fund-raising, and educational needs. For details, write Charisma House Book Group, 600 Rinehart Road, Lake Mary, Florida 32746, or telephone (407) 333-0600.

STEM CELL REVOLUTION by Joseph Christiano, ND, CNC, CNHP
Published by Siloam
Charisma Media/Charisma House Book Group
600 Rinehart Road
Lake Mary, Florida 32746
www.charismahouse.com

Cover design by Justin Evans

Visit the author's website at www.bodyredesigning.com.

Library of Congress Cataloging-in-Publication Data:
An application to register this book for cataloging has been submitted to the Library of Congress.
International Standard Book Number: 978-1-62999-506-9
E-book ISBN: 978-1-62999-507-6

This book contains the opinions and ideas of its author and is based upon sources the author believes to be reliable and current as of the publication date of this book. Some of the views expressed in this book are controversial, and some of the medical opinions describing innovative treatment approaches, while used by a growing number of physicians, are not widely accepted by the medical community. Some aspects of the treatments described are considered complementary, alternative, or integrative medicine (CAIM), and may be the result of clinical understanding and experience rather than controlled clinical research. Readers are encouraged to consult other sources and make independent judgments about the issues discussed.

Neither the publisher nor the author are engaged in rendering professional advice to the individual reader. The ideas, procedures, and protocols contained in this book are solely for informational and educational purposes and should not be regarded as a substitute for professional medical treatment. The nature of your body's health condition is complex and unique. Therefore, you should consult a health professional before you begin any new exercise, nutrition, or supplementation program or if you have questions about your health. Neither the author nor the publisher shall be liable or responsible for any loss or damage allegedly arising from any information or suggestion in this book.

18 19 20 21 22 — 987654321
Printed in the United States of America

MOMENTS WITH MOM

Helen Christiano Guardino
April 1925–September 2017

S PACE ON THIS page could never contain the accolades deserving of this extraordinary woman who lived a vibrant and energetic life between those dates above.

She cared, loved, and raised her four children like a mother hen her chicks. She was a faithful wife to my father, who after fifty-five years of marriage passed away. Then sometime after, she married Mike, my new father for these past eighteen-plus years. She has been a loving and kind mother-in-law with a very close bond with Lori, my wife. She always showed loving-kindness to all her family members. When you met her, you loved her because of her sweet spirit!

To her family she showed her love in so many ways, including her homemade Italian food, bedtime snacks, and immaculate housekeeping. Besides being kindhearted toward everyone, it was her trust in her Savior/Messiah and constant daily prayers for her family that will be forever embedded in my thoughts.

She was my lifetime champion and most energetic cheerleader. She exercised with her pulleys and dumbbells every day, even into her early nineties. She took supplements daily and always clipped health tips from many magazines. Her testimonial/success story that is written in this book is meant to be an inspiration and bring hope to the many people who suffer with kidney disease and diabetes. With our heavenly Father's unmerited favor and her faithful discipline in taking adult stem cell activators, she evaded dialysis and enjoyed living a full life for an additional two and a half years with us.

I told my mom I was dedicating my book to her well before the writing began. Every time I saw her, she would ask if the book was done. But now that the writing is complete, she unexpectedly will never get to see my work in this book.

But her life doesn't end here, for she is where she sent her prayers—with her heavenly Father! For it was those "moments with Mom" and her legacy of caring and love for others that allow me the privilege to carry her torch of compassion and care to my patients and clients everywhere. Though she won't get the chance to see her name in this book, it is her fingerprint that can be found on all the pages, by the one she inspired and whose heart she stole—me!

I love and miss you, Mom, every day!

ETHICAL, ADULT STEM CELL RESEARCH HAS PRODUCED
SOME SIXTY-SEVEN MEDICAL MIRACLES.[1]

—VICE PRESIDENT MIKE PENCE

TABLE OF CONTENTS

ACKNOWLEDGMENTS

THANK YOU, STEVE and Joy Strang and Charisma Media, for this opportunity to present the world with this work about the new "norm" in regenerative medicine—stem cell therapy and activation.

Thank you, Debbie Marrie, my ninja chief editor, for masterfully unscrambling those difficult points I tried to make and crossing all my t's and dotting all my i's with pinpoint accuracy and supersonic speed.

Thank you, Marcos Perez and your awesome staff and sales and marketing team, for sharing my vision.

Thank you, Dr. Makosch, for introducing me to this revolutionary, cutting-edge technology in regenerative medicine—stem cell therapy and PRP therapy. Your expertise and professional knowledge, treating me for all these years, has helped me overcome some of my most painful conditions.

I thank all the people who have placed their trust in my professional expertise and were willing to share their testimonials in this book.

Of course, I thank you, Lori, my wife. You have been the driving force behind me and this work. It has been your love, support, and encouragement through all those years I struggled with chronic pain that helped me overcome being physically handicapped for the rest of my life. I will forever be indebted to you, my love!

Finally I am grateful to my Creator, the God of Abraham, Isaac, and Jacob, who formed me with a design that has all the genetic materials necessary to survive a lifetime. To You I am most grateful and thankful for providing this gift called life and the life to come.

THE GAME CHANGER

I N THIS BOOK, you will learn about stem cells, stem cell treatments, stem cell therapies, and adult stem cell activators and the powerful role they play in optimizing your health. As we delve into this miraculous topic, I want you to view the term *disruptive* as a positive advancement in medicine, science, and nature. Consider *disruptive* as a cutting-edge advancement in both the medical and scientific fields for optimizing the usage of your body's own biological materials to replace conventional medical approaches—adult stem cells.

As you consider the topic of adult stem cell therapy and activators from the standpoint of surpassing the conventional medicine/medical practices with something newer and better, look at it as the game changer.

As technologies and therapies such as adult stem cell therapy and activators continue revolutionizing the way regenerative medicine is conducted, it will be plain to see them as the *new* disruptive technology and therapy in regenerative medicine.

Let me open the world of "disruptive technology" to you by giving you a few examples with the idea of paralleling them with the disruptive technologies in regenerative medicine we'll discuss throughout the book. Once you understand the correlation, I believe you will see there are greater treatments and therapies available today than ever before that will provide you a greater quality of life sooner than later.

What exactly am I talking about? I will try to make this concept as simple as possible, but it will take some open thinking on your part. What I am about to share with you is something you may have never heard of, or it might be something you disagree with or don't believe in—but in any case, it is here and here to stay.

By the way, *disruptive* does not mean something negative but just the opposite. Disruptive technology changes the way in which we do the "norm" by replacing it with a better way, making it the *new* norm—and it always works to our advantage.

So, if you want to ride with me, get a seat on this train now before it pulls out of the station. If not, you will miss seeing where it is headed and all its benefits.

THE GAME CHANGER OF DISRUPTIVE TECHNOLOGY

Right now, as I am writing this book, there are three major disruptive technologies that are presently here, growing at supersonic speed on a global scale. In the very near future, they will change the way you and I conduct our lives.

The three disruptive technologies are blockchain, cryptocurrency, and artificial intelligence (AI).

Let's see what these guys are all about. Please keep in mind, these are real and already disrupting the norm by which people conduct their business in all three areas. Though they are not directly health related, they simply serve as examples of what I mean when I say adult stem cell therapy and activators are the *new* disruptive technology and therapy in regenerative medicine.

But before we look at these three disruptive technologies, let's look at an example of disruptive technology that you may be very familiar with: Uber. I assume you must have heard of Uber by now, but if not, let me explain. Without getting too technical and off base, Uber is a technology platform. The Uber app connects driver-partners and riders. As a driver-partner, you use your own vehicle to pick up riders and drive them to preferred destinations in your city. You're paid a fare for each completed trip. This technology platform creates a peer-to-peer scenario and takes out the middleman, the cab driver service.

Now of course, if you are just a passenger looking for a ride to the airport, then Uber is the perfect fit, primarily because the trip to the airport is less expensive and you save money. Why? Because the middleman has been removed and you are not paying inflated taxi fees.

But if you are a cab driver, your job security may be on the line very soon. You will be replaced! Or worse, if you own the taxicab company, then you are feeling the financial crunch, and if you don't make the right adjustments, your business will soon become a thing of the past. That in a nutshell is what disruptive technology is and does.

THREE EXAMPLES OF DISRUPTIVE TECHNOLOGIES

Blockchain technology

Blockchain technology replaces the way you and I have done our banking for years. In a knockdown version, blockchain allows you to control your money without having to pay the inflated bank fees for services the banking systems force you to pay just to move your money around. By the way, the banking system receives 40 percent of their income from those fees.[1] Who benefits as blockchains become in vogue? We do, because we have a newfound "freedom" with options to move our money as we please without paying the ridiculous, inflated banking fees. What does that do to banking as usual? It makes it obsolete, or at the very least it is now second to the new and improved.

Cryptocurrency

Cryptocurrency—also referred to as "digital currency" or "digital money"—is huge in many parts of the world except here in the United States, but even that is about to change as the evolution of spending money takes on its next stage.

As we look back at the evolution of spending money, we can see how it started when man mined for gold. Then, to spend or buy, he either had to trade gold in exchange for flour or vegetables or have it exchanged at the bank for cash/money. In the same way that gold evolved to fiat money (those dollar bills and coins in your piggy bank) it has now evolved into digital money, i.e., your credit and debit card or technologies such as PayPal. Now the mostly explosive evolutionary stage for buying and spending is cryptocurrency.

Perhaps by now you have heard of Bitcoin, a type of cryptocurrency that has been around since 2008. Cryptocurrency allows you the freedom to send your money to family members who may need an extra buck, or to buy and sell without paying inflated rates and fees or restrictive regulations enforced by who else, the banking system. Your money is protected and cannot be stolen nor is it controlled by any form of controlling agency. It is no longer at the mercy of a few central banking systems' control but tucked safely away in a blockchain that cannot be hacked into. But more so, your money is yours to do with as you please without having to succumb to rigorous banking policies and regulations.

Artificial intelligence

And thirdly, there is AI, or artificial intelligence, which has been in the making for many years. Sure, it may have been unbeknownst to most of us, but it started in the military many years ago. I realize this technology can sound somewhat creepy, but it is here and is moving extremely quickly into our futures. You have heard the rumors of robots replacing humans in the manufacturing scenarios, I'm sure. Well, that is not as futuristic as it may appear. Just in case this disruptive technology platform sounds foreign, there are many current examples of its existence and popularity. I know you have heard about companies called Amazon, Apple, and Facebook. If you've done business with any of them, then you have been familiar with AI technology for some time now, even if you might not have known it.

And of course, you have heard about Siri, right? How about Alexa? I mean, come on, man! Just ask iPhone's Siri or Amazon's Alexa any question or questions you desire. But just to refresh your memory, that pleasant voice you hear from the other side of that electronic device is not a human—it's referred to as "an intelligent personal assistant," or artificial intelligence.

Another example of what disruptive technology does is what happened to a company called Blockbuster. We all remember Blockbuster. After work, everyone would drive to the local Blockbuster video store and rent a movie or two (and I'm sure you also remember VHS technology, which was replaced by DVD technology, which has now been replaced by digital technology). Then within a certain deadline we had to return them to the store or pay an additional fee for being late with the movie(s).

What happened to Blockbuster? It was replaced by a disruptive technology called Netflix. Suddenly, renting a movie became really convenient. Now all you had to do was pay a small monthly fee and simply get online and start streaming unlimited movies of your choice. No driving hassles, no chance of the movie you wanted being unavailable, no late fees, and no tangible DVDs that had to be returned. Netflix provided a better and more convenient means for getting a movie via digital technology, another type of disruptive technology.

Disruptive technology is all around us, and it is the way of the future for all mankind. It will become the new "norm" for doing business as usual in many sectors of society. Whether it is Amazon, Apple, Uber, cryptocurrency, or blockchain technologies, disruptive technology puts an end to doing business as usual, making available an entirely better way for conducting business as usual.

Some people will lose their jobs to robots or other types of AI. Some companies will either get "on the train," so to speak, or lose their business (e.g., Kodak Corporation). The bankers and banking systems worldwide are hustling in preparation for blockchain technology as I write this book.

But in the end, the winners can be you and me if we can embrace disruptive technology. The only thing that will cause you to not benefit like others who have been replaced is if you choose to follow the old or the conventional. To be a winner, simply ask yourself, why should I be held back and limited if there are more freedoms and options for me to choose the means with which I want to conduct and enhance my life, whether it be my livelihood, finances, or even health? As we all embrace disruptive technology, we will find ourselves freed from the limitations of outdated methods/technologies and greatly benefit from the new.

And so it is with your health and well-being through adult stem cell therapy and activators!

IT'S TIME TO JOIN THE REVOLUTION

You may be asking, what exactly is the connection between these disruptive technologies in regenerative medicine and my health? Allow me to connect the dots.

As we can see from the simplified examples of disruptive technologies above, past methods for doing things are being replaced by something revolutionarily newer and better, and this is exactly how it is working when it comes to repairing and healing our bodies from sports injuries, auto accidents, trauma, the aging process, and degenerative illnesses such as diabetes, liver damage, multiple sclerosis, lupus, and heart disease.

You and I have been confined to conventional medicine and its limited practices and protocols for hundreds of years, and there is nothing wrong with that in and of itself. Of course, remedies and modalities have improved over time as man discovered new and more efficient means of healing the body, fighting diseases, and treating various degenerative conditions. Right up to our current day and time there are familiar modalities we use, such as ice and heat therapies, massage therapy, and physical therapy, that play a significant role when an individual is suffering from joint inflammation, injuries, spasms, and strains.

There is the conventional approach taken when facing degenerative diseases and illnesses as well as musculoskeletal problems in orthopedic medicine. The typical or conventional approach is to try some physical therapy, exercise, and then prescribe anti-inflammatory medications and pain medications all as the first line of defense. When all those have run their course, if you are still no better off, then surgery is next in line. You often face a surgery to repair or replace a joint. These treatments and therapies have been around for decades, and they will always be here, but they are slowly losing their attraction and efficacy because the patient is becoming more educated and is in search of more options than the same conventional medical procedures offer today.

The patient of today and the future, particularly the more technologically astute patient, is interested in new technologies and therapies that show greater promise, especially when searching for immediate and long-term improvement. When it comes to wellness, more and more people are learning that they can do what it takes to reach their standard of fitness by themselves using the latest technologies that are available.

Take for example what wearable technology such as the Fitbit watch has done. Today any person can have their own digital wellness program by simply entering some basic personal information like height, weight, and health goals. They can follow a personalized program, track their stats, steps, calories, heart rate, and progress, and never need to pay for another gym membership.

As you and I become more educated and embrace disruptive technologies, we will thrive like we never knew possible. With every new disruptive technology comes more choices or options, which in turn provide greater results.

Whether it is elite professional athletes who are looking for more efficient and rapid ways to repair and recover from injuries so they can return to their sport, or individuals with lingering back pain who need relief so they can return to work to support their families, or the man or woman who has a degenerative condition that needs multiple types of treatments, adult stem cell therapy and activators are two of the new disruptive technologies and therapies in regenerative medicine that will be the game changers for us all. They are revolutionizing the way we think about our health, and that is the reason I've titled this book *Stem Cell Revolution*.

So as you venture throughout this book and learn about stem cell therapies, treatments, and technologies, keep in mind that the world we live in is moving at a supersonic pace. Don't miss your chance to get on board with these new disruptive technologies. I want you to know that there is hope of acquiring quicker healing, faster recovery from injuries, and reversing the negative effects of degenerative diseases. And beyond hope, it is a reality many have begun to experience. Don't get left behind! Join me on the journey to experience the joy of optimum living.

INTRODUCTION

I'M CONSTANTLY AMAZED about the human body and how it provides the means and ways for improving, extending, and taking care of the quality of life for its hosts, you and me. Even after these fifty-plus years of being involved in health, fitness, and naturopathy both personally and professionally, the more I learn and experience about the human body, the more I stand amazed!

If there is one area that fascinates me most, it is how the body provides its own natural genetic elements. These genetic elements or components are responsible for relieving pain, taking down univited viruses and germs, and repairing, restoring, and rejuvenating damaged and diseased tissue. Ultimately, the human body produces enough genetic elements for every man and woman to experience the greatest quality of life, particularly when those genetic elements are better understood and properly applied.

For example, I have experienced more times than I can count how an overweight and unfit body will respond to certain exercise stimuli when taking into account its unique body genetic characteristics. From there, with a little effort, it will transform itself into a symmetrical, hourglass crown winner or a buff, bodybuilding-like physique.

When it comes to improving one's illness profile, I have experienced over and over where an individual's dangerously high cholesterol levels drop down to safe and physiologically ideal levels in just thirty days. Simply by understanding their unique genetic marker—and in this case, their blood type—and making one dietary change like removing a single food type from their diet, the individual greatly improved upon their predetermined genetic illness profile and dodged a potentially health-damaging bullet.

As you may already know, you and I are unique as individuals and yet share many things that make us similar. You and I have our own set of individual and unique genetic markers. These are what set us apart from the pack. These genetic markers are seen in the irises of our eyes, our fingerprints, and our footprints, plus myriad other genetic markers that make us unique and different. Yet within our physical makeup there is something you and I share that makes us rather similar in many ways: cells.

When talking about taking care of the human body, we usually relate to the more obvious and surface-level things such as dietary programs for losing weight, exercise programs for getting fit, or various shapes and sizes of the body. Because we are confronted with sickness, disease, chronic pain, and overall poor health every day of our lives, we tend to see symptoms and turn to symptom stompers—medications—as a form of treatment.

In most conversations about the areas I just mentioned, you don't hear much about the life and duties of the cells in our bodies and the role they play in our day-to-day lives. Granted, it is a complex topic; but if one can be better educated on the functionalities of the cells in our bodies, we will see what miraculous possibilities lie ahead for better health, quicker healing, and faster restoration.

When we better understand what these genetic life-giving elements do to keep the human body functioning normally, you and I will quickly appreciate their value and neccessity. The human body is the most complex and masterfully created design and network of cells, all with unique functions and duties, and it must be understood if one plans on living a healthy, disease-free life.

Since all of mankind have cells, let's explore their different functions and how they impact the best quality of our physical lives. I dare not attempt to fill these pages with the names and types of cells, their structures and duties found throughout the entire makeup of our bodies. But be assured our physiological makeup and bodily functions are only possible by the health and efficacy of our cells and how they can rejuvenate and repair and produce optimum life within us.

In fact, should our seven to nine pounds of skin be removed, there beneath would be found trillions and trillions of cells all working in concert with one another—unless something causes them to malfunction or lose their ability to perform their duties.

Therefore, to keep this book concise and on point, I have chosen to bypass the almost enumerable amount of different types of cellular structures and their functions and instead focus on specific cells that are found in every tissue throughout your body and mine: *adult stem cells!*

As you read through this book, I will be the messenger of insights for you. Though I am not a physician who specializes in stem cell procedures, therapies, and treatments, I do have a vast knowledge of the topic both personally and professionally. As we venture through the book, I will share my personal experiences in dealing with chronic pain and the relief I received from stem cell therapy and treatments.

We will learn about when stem cell therapy came about and how it has evolved from the very highly controversial embryonic stem cell technology to becoming "the new norm" in regenerative and orthopedic medicine—adult stem cell therapies. We will see how powerful these adult stem cells are and how stem cell therapy can treat other conditions such as Crohn's disease, cancer, multiple sclerosis (MS), liver disorders, heart conditions, lung problems, and many more.

Stem cell therapy is so "disruptive" in the world of regenerative medicine that it has made conventional medicine approaches to musculoskeletal problems look outdated and ineffective. This cutting-edge therapy is so efficacious, people from all walks of life are taking advantage of it, from well-known global sports figures such as Tiger Woods (PGA Golf) and Fred Couples (PGA Golf) to NFL football players and NBA basketball players. But stem cell therapy is not only for the elite athletes of the world. Today, like never before, the not-so-high-profile person is embracing these new technologies and treatments. Many who are facing possible joint repair or replacement surgery or who have been living with chronic pain or degenerative illnesses are now finding relief from pain and restoration from poor health conditions.

Our adult stem cells are our bodies' natural repair crews. When they are performing at their optimum, the damaged cells found in tissues throughout our bodies are quickly repaired and restored. That is why we can recover from an injury or sickness or trauma. But what happens when these "repair crews" get damaged, when they can no longer function optimally and cannot repair the tissue and cells in our bodies like they do normally? What do we do in that case?

Later in the book I will discuss in detail how you and I can rejuvenate and repair our own adult stem cells that are not able to do their cellular repair work. You will learn how to "activate" your own stem cells so they return to optimum function and perform their regular duties—*cellular communication or signalling.*

Since there are specific adult stem cells for every tissue and cell in our bodies—for the kidneys, liver, lungs, heart, gallbladder, ligaments and tendons, peripheral nerves, central nervous system, and so on—it is easy to understand the importance and value of adult stem cell activation.

You will be introduced to twenty-six targeted adult stem cell activators and the specific areas they target for repair and rejuvenation. Perhaps you will identify with some of these areas of concern that you may be dealing with at this present time.

We will hear from many people who share their testimonials about their experience using adult stem cell activators and what I would like to refer to as their "miraculous" results!

Besides learning about stem cells and the treatments and therapies that are available for you today and the many benefits that come from stem cell activation, we all need to factor in our lifestyles.

It goes without saying, the type of foundation or base on which you decide to build your future makes all the difference when it comes to success or failure—and without a doubt, this applies to your health. It doesn't matter if you are using conventional medicine for treatments, exploring cutting-edge stem cell therapies and treatments, or going all natural with alternative and naturopathy remedies and protocols—your lifestyle should include major components of recovery and prevention.

I will share with you some very helpful and practical healthy lifestyle practices that include the importance of establishing a psychological and nutritional base. Hopefully, when you're done reading this book, you'll have a better understanding of how and what to do to:

- Slow down the negative effects of the aging process

- Improve your illness profile

- Lose weight

- Live pain-free, and more!

We'll explore the concepts of making food choices based on your genetics, the value of hormonal balance, and reducing illness while enhancing a vibrant life. You will see the important benefits of exercise and how it keeps you in good health and form as you age, plus what dietary supplements you should consider as a means of supplementing your nutrient intake from the foods you eat.

I believe as you delve into my book, you will discover so much more about yourself and the amazing God-given genetic materials you have at your disposal and how they will make all the difference in living your life at the optimum level possible.

SECTION I

Adult Stem Cells— Disruptive Technology

Y OU'RE ABOUT TO start reading section 1, where I'll lay the foundation for understanding this new disruptive technology that harnesses the power of your very own stem cells. We'll examine the basics about stem cells, the body's remodeling and repair crew. We'll take a brief look at the history of stem cell research, outline the types of stem cells and some key terminology you need to understand, and discover which kinds of stem cells are the most widely researched in association with tissue repair.

I'll also share some of my own personal journey with pain that led me to discover more about the amazing things stem cells can do, and I'll introduce you to someone very special to me whose experience with stem cell activators stands as a testimony to the improved quality of life they can provide.

My goal is to provide you with groundbreaking information that can open your eyes to a whole new world of treatment opportunities you might not have known about before now. And I want you to start feeling better as soon as possible, so let's get started!

CHAPTER 1

WHAT ARE STEM CELLS?

A s I MENTIONED in the preface of this book, right before our
eyes we are experiencing a form of "disruptive" technology and
therapy in regenerative medicine like never before. But before
we learn about this disruptive technology involving adult stem cells,
their unique functions, the multiple areas of the body they can help
repair and/or rebuild, and all the miraculous results that come from
the various stem cell treatments and therapies available, I need to make
a quick statement to clarify my position on the use of embryonic stem
cells extracted from aborted unborn fetuses.

Embryonic stem cell treatment or therapy (different than cord stem
cells that have been extracted from the umbilical cord *after* the birth of a
child) has been a huge, controversial topic for many people for many years.

I have always believed that bioethics must be taken into consideration
and even challenged whenever science and medicine begin tampering
with the human body for research or any noble cause. New scientific
findings and medical technological advancements with cutting-edge
treatments when dealing with the human body have (and probably
always will) aroused suspicion, doubt, and certainly controversy, and
I believe that's as it should be. Embryonic stem cell treatment and
therapy where the stem cells have been extracted from aborted fetuses
is no different.

So as one who embraces the sanctity of life, it would be a major con-
flict of my belief and conscientiousness to accept the medical procedure
of terminating (murdering/killing) a fetus for the sake of science and
medical advancement. Since I come into agreement with the medical

research that supports life beginning upon conception, that precious fetus is, to me, a human life. This creation of life living within the womb of its mother is deserving of protection and equal human rights, and is entitled to the opportunity of growing up into an adult.

I therefore cannot support nor justify the usage of aborted fetus embryonic stem cells. This part of stem cell research and treatment is unacceptable for the sake of improving mankind's state of health or scientific and medical advancements, despite the nobility of intent.

In my humble opinion, the acceptable standard should not be determined by scientific and medical data or intent alone but should ultimately be determined by the standard of the highest judge—the Creator of the fetus!

THE HISTORY OF STEM CELL RESEARCH

Just read a sports magazine such as *Sports Illustrated* or a science magazine such as *Discover*, or print advertisements or even TV specials, and it won't be long until the topic of stem cell therapy and treatments appears.

It is becoming commonplace to read about world-class professional athletes who are turning to stem cell and/or PRP (platelet-rich plasma) treatments as the new norm for healing and repairing injuries instead of conventional medicine. But stem cell therapy is not just for the elite.

Everyday people are also taking full advantage of these latest cutting-edge medical treatments—people who have been involved in auto accidents and suffer from spinal and joint injuries, or people who suffer from chronic pain, degenerative illnesses, and multiple health issues. Even people like myself who have benefited from several of these disruptive treatments and therapies have discovered this new norm as a better and more efficacious means of practicing regenerative medicine.

We can go back as far as the mid-1800s to see where stem cell research began. At that time research taught us that certain cells had the capability to differentiate, or change, into other cells. Unfortunately, it was the early stages of stem cell research, when embryonic stem cells were extracted from the termination of unborn fetuses, that got all the bad press—and rightfully so.

I'm sure if you, like most people, have heard anything about stem cell therapy and research, you most likely have associated aborted fetuses with this breakthrough in regenerative medicine. Like many, you were probably in total opposition to anything that had to with stem cell therapy.

But many who have followed its progression over the years have found out that stem cell therapy and research have made some very amazing strides. As continued research and scientific discoveries have been made, we have found out that stem cell therapy and treatments are available in multiple applications—and, the great news is, without using stem cells from terminated unborn fetuses. Allow me to move us along with this understanding and show when and where things have advanced in this disruptive therapy in regenerative medicine since the beginning of its journey.

In the early 1900s, attempts were made to fertilize mammalian eggs outside of the human body, where the discovery was made that some cells had the capacity to generate blood cells. Later, around 1968, the first successful bone marrow transplant was performed. The following are several milestones in stem cell research:

- 1978—Discovery of stem cells in human cord blood

- 1981—Development of first in vitro stem cell line from mice

- 1988—Creation of embryonic stem cell lines from a hamster

- 1995—Researchers derive embryonic stem cell line from a primate

- 1997—Lamb cloned from stem cells

- 1997—Leukemia origin found as hematopoietic stem cells indicating possible proof of cancer stem cells

- 1999–2000—Scientists produce different stem cells in mice, leading to the discovery that cells from bone marrow can produce liver or nerve cells and even the brain can produce other cells.

- 2005—Scientists discover that the umbilical cord has unique stem cells referred to as embryonic-like stem cells. All this leads to greatest heights for cell-based therapies.

- 2007—Scientists discover a new stem cell in amniotic fluid which eventually proves to be a viable alternative to embryonic stem cells.[1]

As we see the history of stem cell therapy, treatment, and research abound and advance through the years, there are also many new discoveries and multiple types of treatments becoming the new norm. With any new treatments and applications should come safety policies and standards.

WHERE IS STEM CELL TECHNOLOGY TODAY?

There is no doubt that stem cell therapies and treatments are continually advancing. I say "advancing" because I do not see it slowing down anytime soon. Based on my professional associations with stem cell physicians and scientists and from their experiences and newly gained knowledge, it is obvious that stem cell treatments will be here well into the future.

Stem cell therapy is being used to treat many more health conditions today than back in the day of its infancy. From my own personal experiences as a stem cell patient and advocate, I see it becoming the treatment of choice in regenerative and orthopedic medicine as well as in the treatment of many degenerative diseases.

Today, stem cell therapies have advanced to such levels that they can be implemented to treat crippling and debilitating conditions such as spinal cord injuries, kidney disease, diabetes, heart disease, cancer, and orthopedic and musculoskeletal conditions.

Speaking of orthopedic medicine, I dare to make the claim that eventually stem cell therapy is going to be the new norm in orthopedic medicine! Let me explain why I call this daring. Even in our current day and time, should you have an inflamed and painful knee, your physician's prognosis is not going to be all that hopeful and will certainly be limited to what can be accomplished. Typically you would be given prescriptions that cover a multiplicity of treatments: anti-inflammatories, painkillers, some physical therapy, and perhaps chiropractic work. That is just to treat your painful symptoms. But you and I know the outcome of that medical process—over time you would experience no improvement, less mobility, more pain, continual swelling, and life would become more challenging.

And worse, should your diagnosis be a bone-on-bone scenario (meaning your joint has degenerated to the point that bone is rubbing against bone), then you would be left with absolutely no alternative treatments, no options but to get a second opinion if you so decided to choose one. After all that, a prognosis for knee replacement surgery would be handed down to you—until now! Today's stem cell treatments are so advanced that in a few hours as an outpatient, you can have a minimally invasive procedure done by simply injecting your own stem cells into the knee joint. It may take only one or possibly several treatments, but over time the knee will begin growing back new cartilage. That bone-on-bone death sentence will become last night's news, and you will get a whole new grip on living life to its fullest.[2]

Worldwide Stem Cell Research

Just a few brief words about stem cell research throughout the world.

- Many countries throughout the world have conducted and are conducting stem cell research. Some of them are the United States, Germany, Switzerland, Spain, Italy, Canada, Australia, Austria, and South Korea.

- Governing policies and laws per individual country can vary. For example, countries like Canada seem to be more flexible in the field of stem cell research. Whereas the European Union does not fund research that results in embryonic destruction, the United States funds embryonic stem cell research, though the funds are limited.

- Each country with its different political, governmental laws and ethical standards can positively affect the other countries as this field of adult stem cell research continues to prove its efficacious results and therapeutic potential.[3]

WHAT ARE STEM CELLS?

Maybe you've heard of stem cells on television, but you aren't sure what they are or the role they play with regards to your overall health and state of well-being. If so, don't be discouraged. My goal here is to present this highly scientific and medically advanced topic using a non-scientific approach so as to make this topic more palatable.

Let's start with understanding our cells. A cell is a unit of life that is basic in function and structure. Did you know that you and I are made up of trillions of these little guys? From a more scientific and cellular perspective, you and I would be considered "multicellular." Our total existence is dependent upon our cells, whether we need energy to carry out simple daily tasks and recreational activities or more strenuous activities such as sports or heavy physical workloads like construction work. Also, don't forget about the assimilating and digesting of nutrients from the food and beverages we consume. This multitrillion-cell network is directly correlated to everything we do in life. Keeping the cells healthy and functioning is key to everyone's overall health, youthfulness, and quality of life.

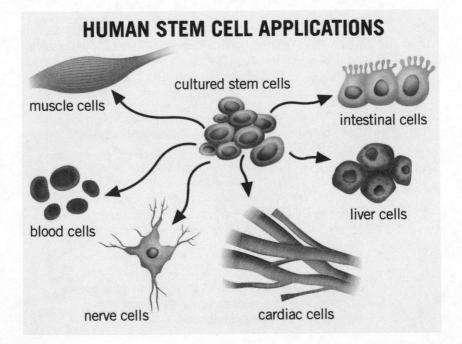

HUMAN STEM CELL APPLICATIONS

muscle cells

cultured stem cells

intestinal cells

blood cells

liver cells

nerve cells

cardiac cells

There are more than two hundred different cell types in the human body, each with specialized and very different functions. But there is a special group of cells in the body that come from a simpler type of cell that is not specialized. These unspecialized cells are the stem cells. They are basically cells that don't yet have a specific job in the body. Stem cells are *unspecialized*, meaning they can reproduce themselves by dividing and under the right conditions are able to become cells with specialized jobs, such as nerve, kidney, or heart stem cells. To put it another way, stem cells have two interesting characteristics:

1. Replication/self-renewal

Adult stem cells can replicate, or multiply, themselves. This replication factor contributes to enhancing their ability for rapid healing and recovery.

2. Differentiation

Stem cells can turn into, or become, other types of cells, such as pancreas or liver cells, in which case they would take on the specific functions of pancreas cells or liver cells. This amazing phenomenon occurs after the stem cell divides during the first few days of life.

In the early embryo development stages, a cluster of less than fifty cells multiplies into hundreds of uniquely specialized cells and assume the roles they play in nature's normal preparation process for adult life, survival, and existence. As the fetus grows, some stem cells become skin, some become heart tissue, and others become the rest of the organs. Eventually, these embryonic stem cells disappear. An adult body no longer contains cells that can generate any kind of cell—at least not in the natural course of life. (Through research, scientists have learned how to cause adult stem cells to become other types of cells, and that's what this book is about.)

But after the embryonic stem cells disappear, other types of stem cells remain in the body. Some of these adult stem cells will eventually be destroyed by illness, injuries, and even the aging process.

Stem cells are the body's cellular remodeling and repair crew.

Yes, our adult stem cells are vulnerable to the aging process. Unfortunately, as we age, the production of our stem cells diminishes. Our stem cells are usually created and distributed from our bone marrow, but over time the marrow production decreases and it no longer releases as many stem cells as it once did. This reduction in systemic circulation of stem cells throughout our body is the main reason nagging injuries and illnesses take much longer to heal. It is not just because we are getting older, but rather a combination of the aging process, exposure to environmental toxins, injuries, disease, and other negative factors that is the culprit. The reality is, having fewer stem cells in our bodies means fewer cells are available for repairing and rejuvenating our bodies naturally.[4] (Later, in section 2, you will learn how the adult stem activators come to the rescue and rejuvenate and repair certain types of stem cells that are destroyed through injury, disease, or age.)

Stem Cells 101

One of the most interesting and fascinating phenomena about the human body is that every human being on planet Earth—regardless of our genetic and physiological differences, age, gender, race, creed, religion, or socio-economic status—has adult stem cells. These stem cells were given to us at birth and are a part of our genetic makeup.

The most simplified and basic job description that I could give you is that *stem cells are the body's cellular remodeling and repair crew.* Adult stem cells repair damaged cells naturally to best support life, provide optimum health, and counterpunch diseases for every man and woman.

There are many varieties of stem cells serving different purposes in your body's hugely complex system to keep you healthy, resilient, and able to survive. Here is a quick list of several types of stem cells and related terminology so you can get better acquainted with the topic.

- **Stem cells**—Cells that can divide and self-renew for an indefinite period to differentiate into specialized cells. Stem cells are found in bone marrow, blood, and adipose tissue (body fat). The greatest number of stem cells, by the millions, are found in adipose, or fat tissue.

- **Adult stem cells**—Also referred to as *somatic* cells, adult stem cells include any stem cell other than an egg or sperm cell in the female or male, respectively. Somatic stem cells are an increasingly used source of stem cells derived from adult tissues such as bone marrow, blood, fat, and other organs. Less potent than embryonic stem cells, somatic cells have a more limited number of cell types into which they can differentiate.

- **Embryonic stem cells**—Stem cells capable of dividing for a long period of time without differentiation. These stem cells are derived from preimplantation embryos and have been the subject of much debate in medical bioethics. Due to their primitive (undifferentiated) nature, they can lead to the creation of many cell types, which may cause problems if implanted in living tissue without careful control. Embryonic stem cell use is very controversial in many religious, societal, and cultural circles, and I do not condone this practice.

- **Cord blood stem cells**—Stem cells present in the umbilical cord blood that can be collected after birth and stored for later use in therapeutic treatment. Cord blood stem cells are hematopoietic (they can produce blood cells) and are commonly used to treat cancer patients who have undergone chemotherapy. Hematopoietic stem cells form the red and white blood cells and platelets, and they are found in bone marrow and umbilical cord blood.

- **Mesenchymal stem cells**—The current, somewhat general term for non-blood somatic (adult) stem cells from a variety of tissues in the body.

- **Autologous transfer**—Transfer of adult stem cells to a different location in the same person. The transplant of stem cells to different areas of the same body carries little risk of the resulting tissue being rejected.

- **Differentiation**—Cell differentiation is the result of the interaction between a cell's genes and the external environment, including physical and chemical conditions. The cell can differentiate into specialized cells such as those of the liver, heart, or bone.

  Various techniques have been devised to cause a cell to differentiate into specific cell types for therapeutic purposes by influencing the signaling pathways of proteins on the cell's external surface; this is known as directed differentiation.

- **Multipotent**—A stem cell can be multipotent in that it has the ability to differentiate into a number of different cell types in the body, such as blood cells, bone cells, or cartilage cells.

- **Regenerative medicine**—A general term describing the use of stem cells differentiated to form specific cell types in repairing or replacing damaged cells or tissues.

MESENCHYMAL STEM CELLS

Mesenchymal stem cells (MSCs) are the most popularly applied and researched adult stem cells in association with cellular and tissue repair in the musculoskeletal system. These stem cells are found and extracted from adipose tissue (body fat), skin, and bone marrow, and can differentiate into other mesenchymal stem cells, such as soft tissue like ligaments and tendons, bone, muscle, fibroblasts, and adipose tissue. This is their signature marker that makes them different and unique from other types of stem cells.

When oxygen and blood flow to certain areas of the body is extremely limited or even nonexistent, the body does not get enough of these repair cells (MSCs) to the damaged or injured area. Common areas in the body that don't receive much oxygen flow, or are in a state of hypoxia, include our joints, meniscus tissue, ligaments, tendons, and rotator cuffs. But through new stem cell treatments, MSCs can be targeted to these areas in your body that do not heal well on their own. That is why stem cells and the use of stem cell therapy can prevent unnecessary orthopedic surgeries and surgical procedures.

A study titled "Current Concepts: The Role of Mesenchymal Stem

Cells in the Management of Knee Osteoarthritis" concluded that MSCs have the "potential for improving function and decreasing inflammation" in the joints of animals, which may be able to transfer over into human patients.[5] This type of research continues to flourish as experts learn more about the use of stem cells in the body and the best ways to apply them for healing.

Since stem cells have the unique ability to develop into other types of cells and tissues, they have been successfully utilized to heal the body in unprecedented ways. There are numerous benefits to using stem cell therapy in place of more invasive options like joint replacement surgery. More than anything else, stem cell treatment is highly sought after because it can reduce pain, increase range of motion, and accelerate healing in a simple yet effective manner. Stem cells are harvested and then administered to the site of injury using a quick injection. The joints and body do not have to endure a difficult recovery period or risk implant rejection. Instead, progress steadily strengthens over the span of weeks and months until the treated area of the body feels nearly like new!

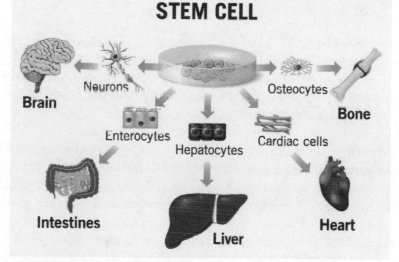

Mesenchymal stem cells are also being used for heart tissue repair after a patient has experienced a myocardial infarction (heart attack), as well as Crohn's disease, diabetes, kidney dysfunction, and other illnesses. Imagine someone who has had a heart attack. After the patient endures a horrifying trip to the hospital, the doctors' first line of defense is to try and stabilize the patient as best they can. But the cellular damage to the heart cells is irreparable, which consequently becomes a precursor for or places the person at high risk for additional medical problems. But what if the damage to heart cells could be reversed?

Doctors at the University of Miami Miller School are working on new therapies that can address this condition. By extracting stem cells from bone marrow, the damage to heart cells can be reversed. With advanced stem cell therapies like these, the surviving heart attack patient can have much more hope for living with a greater quality of life.

For additional reading on stem cell therapy and heart attacks, here are a few resources that explain in greater detail:

- Boyle, Andrew J., Steven P. Schulman, and Joshua M. Hare. "Stem Cell Therapy for Cardiac Repair: Ready for the Next Step." *Circulation* 114 (2006): 339–52. http://dx.doi.org/10.1161/CIRCULATIONAHA.105.590653.

- Laflamme, M. A. and C. E. Murry. "Regenerating the Heart." *Nature Biotechnology* 23, no. 7 (July 2005): 845–56. https://doi.org/10.1038/nbt1117.

- Zimmet, J. M. and J. M. Hare. "Emerging Role for Bone Marrow Derived Mesenchymal Stem Cells in Myocardial Regenerative Therapy." *Basic Research in Cardiology* 100, no. 6 (November 2005): 471–81. https://doi.org/10.1007/s00395-005-0553-4.

With these types of clinical tests and trials, we can only anticipate a greater potential for repairing damaged cells from other bodily systems and organs such as the liver, lungs, spinal cord, and pancreas (for diabetes). As stem cell research and treatment continues, I believe the sky will be the limit for rapidly healing and repairing common ailments, diseases, and chronic pain. Stem cell therapy is superseding—and will continue to supersede—our present-day treatments of medications and surgical procedures.

THE SIGNIFICANCE OF STEM CELLS

Since you and I are made up of trillions of cells, both specialized and unspecialized (stem cells), doesn't it make sense to learn everything we can about ourselves to be best prepared for illness and injury, healing and recovery, and longevity and quality of life?

If we are planning on living long, healthy lives, it would behoove us to take note that this will not happen unless we are prudent with what we have been given to work with. Genetically speaking, each of us has been given just so much clay to work with, and it is our responsibility to make the most of what we have been given. My motto is, "Being a faithful caretaker of your health is not an option but an obligation!"

The chance of developing cancer, Crohn's disease, MS, diabetes, kidney disease, and many other serious degenerative health conditions is constantly growing throughout one's lifetime. Stem cells are significant because they are already being used to treat these health conditions and more. To me, it only stands to reason that the more scientific and medical stem cell research is done, with continual study and testing plus advancements in treatment and therapies, the greater our possibilities for overcoming disease, illness, chronic pain, and injuries. The results will be manifested by a greater quality of life for you and me, as well as our children and grandchildren.

What if researchers could identify why cells become cancerous and how it could be prevented? Or what if they discovered a natural way to counterpunch these degenerating and even terminal conditions with stem cell therapies and without the use of chemotherapy and radiation treatments? Wouldn't that be significant enough to cause you to have more of an interest in learning what is available for you or your loved one facing such dilemmas?

---

*Being a faithful caretaker of your health
is not an option but an obligation!*

Think about the waiting lists for organ donations. Folks who experience such health conditions are overwhelmed and challenged physically, emotionally, and financially day by day in the waiting phase for an organ donor. Sadly enough, many patients expire before they get a transplant. (See section 2 to read a patient's testimony about how they were able to be removed from a kidney transplant waiting list.)

Amazingly, these areas of the body mentioned above have the possibility of being repaired and rebuilt without the use of medications, foreign materials, and/or invasive surgical reconstruction. You and I naturally possess this genetic treasure chest of adult stem cells and can enjoy a better quality of life simply by using our God-given genetic materials.

Because stem cells are unspecialized, they can grow new bone tissue, cartilage, organs, nerves, breasts for a cancer reconstruction patient, and even muscle tissue that has been damaged or torn. The medical and scientific communities have been revolutionized by the advancements in stem cell therapy. Stem cell research has significantly expanded in recent years as scientists and medical experts seek to uncover the true extent of the power of stem cells to heal the body. This is especially true when it comes to musculoskeletal conditions like joint pain.

According to biomedical engineers at Johns Hopkins University like Jennifer Elisseeff, PhD, "We've already used adult stem cells to create tissue resembling cartilage…we think we've come up with a clinically practical way to deliver the cells to the site of an injury, where they can grow to replace injured bone or cartilage."[6]

Stem cells and stem cell treatments are clearly disruptive by providing the most advanced technological therapies that surpass all conventional applications. Adult stem cell technology is an intriguing and promising area of science and medicine. I can attest personally to being treated for certain orthopedic conditions, so I am not just speaking theoretically. There is no doubt in my mind that should you be diagnosed as needing some orthopedic surgical procedure, you will wish you had access to some stem cell scientist or physician who could spare you the horrifying experience of undergoing a possibly unnecessary surgery. We can all benefit from learning more details about what stem cells are and how they can improve our lives.

BENEFITS OF USING STEM CELLS TO HEAL THE BODY

I realize that for most people the topic of stem cells, stem cell research, and stem cell therapy can be a little challenging—not to mention a bit foreign and misunderstood. Obviously, when misunderstood, it can cause a litany of questions, doubts, and apprehensions. For many the big concern is the termination of the life of a fetus just for the purpose and intent of advancing the quality of life for others—I get it! I condemn that practice, and it is not what this book is about.

Please hang in there with me, because there is a much larger picture of what stem cell therapy can do for you and me. Adult stem cells can be isolated or extracted from certain areas of one's own body (without involving embryonic stem cells from a terminated fetus), and this fact should be encouraging and help you let your guard down, so to speak. My goal is to educate you on the topic of adult stem cells and adult stem cell therapy so that you feel confident about the legitimacy and ethical soundness of this medical phenomenon.

I hope all this information excites you like it does me. It has been my lifelong passion to find treatment answers for people who, maybe like yourself, have lost hope for finding remedies to recover from chronic pain, inflammatory conditions, or major health events; who are seeking alternatives to knee replacements, hip replacements, or other surgeries; and who wish there were answers to their questions.

We are living in a time unlike one hundred, fifty, forty, thirty, and even twenty years ago, when the chances of restoring damaged tissue or repairing a joint was nothing more than a trial and error, coin-toss game. As the scientific and medical communities continue in this world of stem cell research, stem cell therapies, and cutting-edge technological advancements, every man and woman now and in the future will have the ability to live healthy and normal lives by using the God-given adult stem cells within them. Now let's consider the concept of stem cell therapy and learn about the various applications of usage from our own stem cells.

CHAPTER 2

ADULT STEM CELL THERAPY OPTIONS

ADULT STEM CELL treatments are valid and efficacious; many top professional athletes use stem cell treatments to rebuild and repair the injured areas of their joints so they can get back to their sports in record time. As I mentioned in the opening of this book, stem cell treatment is the "disruptive" treatment and therapy of the twenty-first century!

Reading all about stem cells, stem cell research, and stem cell therapy/ treatments is very educational if you have an interest in the topic. But when you or someone you know is the one living with the day-to-day misery of inflamed and painful joints, this information is a life changer. Perhaps this is you and you've been living out each day with grueling pain and discomfort, embracing that old mind-set that you just have to "suck it up." My friend, I'm here to tell you this is not living. Trust me—I know too well what it is like to live with chronic pain.

My passion is to help people be healthier! I am passionate about being a messenger of hope and promise for a better, healthier body. Even as I write this book, I am still in pursuit of more remedies, protocols, and modalities that help individuals like you find the right treatment or stem cell therapy that will relieve or even eliminate chronic pain so you can return to living a pain-free life as it was meant to be enjoyed.

Along with further educating you on this miraculous topic regarding its history and advancements over the years in research, trials, and actual treatments, I also chose to include several of my personal experiences with this technology. After all, what better way can I attest to the efficacy of these treatments than to share my very own experiences?

MY FIRST STEM CELL TREATMENT

Back in September 2008, much had been going on in my personal life and in my business—all in a positive, productive way—but life was very busy. In fact, it was at that precise time that my wife, Lori, and I finished a lengthy process of merging our business and personal lives into our new home and business location. Even though a couple of years had gone by, the domino effect of the move eventually took its toll in a big way on my lower back.

It had been approximately twenty years since I'd had emergency lumbar back surgery in the late '80s. Oh, I responded very well to the surgery, and within twenty-three hours I was home performing therapy and rehab. Over the next two decades, I did everything I had done before the surgery, which included operating my personal training business, doing my own personal weight training, jogging, snow skiing, and golfing—everything. But twenty years and a lot of physical activities later, my back seemed to reach its breaking point. (I think the heavy-duty furniture that Lori thought I could move into the new house was the straw that literally broke my back.)

That's when I started experiencing constant lower back pain, particularly sciatica, or nerve pain. At first I would ice it, then heat it, then heat it *and* ice it. I also did floor stretches to free up the nerve and loosen the muscles every day. But the level of pain grew more and more intense to the point that my everyday activities, which were many, were becoming a struggle for me.

The pain was constant and intense, so I thought I would see my family physician about doing something to relieve the pain. Now I found myself on anti-inflammatories, which never took the pain away and at best barely masked the pain. I was miserable every day. As is the usual progression when someone is dealing with degenerative musculoskeletal (joint and muscle) pain, I was prescribed pain medication. All of this was going contrary to my personal and professional belief in natural health remedies. But I could hardly function and needed some relief so I could still live my day-to-day life.

During this time I was asked to be a featured guest speaker at a health and wellness function in Hot Springs, Arkansas. I had become so incapacitated from the excruciating pain that I could hardly walk. Now I could feel pain not only running down my leg but also in my hips. The thought of a five-hour round-trip flight, three days of walking around a convention center, and speaking center stage on the topic of health and wellness was freaking me out mentally on top of the physical pain.

The weekend passed, and Lori and I were on the plane flying back home. During the flight Lori noticed an ad in one of the flight magazines. The headline didn't say much—just something simple like "Arthritis." As she read it carefully, she noticed that it referred to a clinic in Miami, Florida, just a few hours from us.

After we returned home, Lori set an appointment for me to go to the clinic in the ad and meet a physician who specialized in stem cell therapy. At that time I had only heard about stem cells and treatments through some medical journals and had never actually had a treatment done to me.

We drove to the Center for Regenerative Medicine clinic in North Miami for my initial consultation and treatment. I was hardly able to sit in the chair due to the pain—I needed some relief! I was both a little nervous and excited at the same time as this was going to be a totally new experience for me.

The doctor began to explain what stem cells did and how he would extract them and inject them into my lower/lumbar back. After he reviewed my MRIs and physical examination, the stem cell procedure began.

The first phase was to have a blood draw. Then the blood was spun in a centrifuge. The process separated the plasma and growth factors and stem cells. After thirty minutes or so, that procedure was complete. Then he had me lie facedown on a bed, where he began injecting what he called the "medicine" (which was nothing more than my own stem cells and blood components) into my L-5 and S-1 lumbar joints, or spinal column.

As he injected the stem cells, I felt pressure but no real pain. The entire injecting of my stem cells took about five minutes. From there he had me sit up and walk over to another room, where I was wrapped up in heating blankets for about thirty minutes. After that I was consulted on what to expect and was sent home. The entire process took around four hours.

At the end of his final consultation that day he mentioned that perhaps I should call him in a couple of months to follow up and see how I was doing. We drove three and a half hours back home, and to my amazement I had zero pain or discomfort. I wasn't sure what to expect other than what he'd said, but ultimately he said I could go back to normal living.

November rolled around, and as usual Lori and I were busy with family plans for Thanksgiving and running the business. The crazy thing was that since my stem cell treatment in September a couple of months earlier, I noticed that I wasn't having much (if any) pain in my lower back, so I didn't feel the need for a second treatment.

But in February 2009, I unfortunately started feeling the daily back pain return, so I scheduled a second stem cell treatment. This time it took two treatments because my back condition was complicated due to the emergency back surgery I'd had twenty years previously and what I was dealing with currently.

Let me say this as a precaution, should you ever decide to have a surgical procedure: When your body naturally heals itself from wounds—in this case, having my back cut open—it grows scar tissue. Everyone will have to deal with scar tissue at some point down the road. Blood and oxygen cannot flow into scar tissue, but it continues to grow, and only another surgical procedure can remove it.

The problem I was having was the scar tissue growth from my back surgery twenty years earlier, which was now encroaching or impinging the nerves in my back. In addition to the scar tissue buildup I had four bulging discs and moderate stenosis that were all contributing to the painful neuropathy, or nerve pain.

This time my doctor recommended that we increase the treatment by adding more stem cells for the treatment, which he collected by performing a mini liposuction procedure on my stomach. The procedure, which was a first for me, was not at all painful. It was not a cosmetic procedure (sorry, ladies); he simply removed approximately 60–100 ccs of adipose tissue, or belly fat. From the adipose tissue he extracted millions more stem cells than were taken from the blood.

After thirty to forty-five minutes of preparing the blood components and stem cells in the lab, the doctor loaded the syringes. I lay facedown, and he injected the stem cells into my lower back joints just as he had done in the initial treatment, except this treatment was loaded with more stem cells.

After the protocol was through, he sent me home and told me to come back for a second treatment. As I mention many times, since every one of us is different, our conditions may also be different, so therefore every one of us will respond differently. The results of any stem cell treatment will vary because there are several variables to consider, such as age, healing and recovery ability, and severity of the condition. In my case, my back problem was complicated. After getting back home, it was life as usual—but this time, without any pain. I was pain-free for several more years.

STEM CELL INJECTIONS

Stem cell injections, or platelet injections, allow stem cells to grow into and even multiply cartilage tissue in the joints, saving a patient from unnecessary types of medical surgical procedures like knee or hip replacements. There was a time when a bone-on-bone joint condition was next to a death sentence of the joint. Now that same joint can be rejuvenated with PRP (platelet-rich plasma) and stem cells and have new cartilage growth providing the protection between the bones it once had when healthy.

The beauty is that this procedure is all-natural with no side effects and requires no dangerous additives, chemicals, or medications. Therefore, there is no toxicity in the body and no concern for rejection as it is just the individual's own blood and components.

Each individual case is different and results will vary, but it generally takes two to three months for the repair process to take place, although noticeable improvement can be experienced well before that.

Experiencing a stem cell treatment is quite unique. It sounds like it would be a very invasive procedure and require an overnight stay in the hospital, but not so. It only takes a few hours for a stem cell treatment consisting of a blood draw, mini liposuction, injections to a single site or sites, and some physical therapy. It is an outpatient procedure, and you are sent home the same day.

To me, stem cell therapy and treatments have been the most effective treatments I have experienced—and I have had many other different types of regenerative treatments. This is truly the wave of the future for restoring health.

STEM CELL INFUSIONS/IV

With the popularity of this "disruptive" stem cell therapy growing among orthopedic and medical physicians and practitioners around the world, the topic of injecting stem cells intravenously is gaining much popularity. The procedure and purpose of stem cell IV (intravenous) injections is different than that of injecting stem cells into a degenerated joint or site.

When stem cells are injected into a location or site such as the knee joint or hip joint—or in my case, the back—the pinpoint accuracy of the injection to the exact location of the damaged area in the joint is most critical and can be accomplished by using ultrasound for guidance. The use of ultrasound and a monitor screen allows the practitioner to see exactly where the injection is going. However, when stem cells are administered via intravenous injections, the stem cells are free to roam throughout the body. This systemic approach to new tissue growth and repair makes some of the incurable cases curable, and it can access hard-to-reach areas in the body.

For these reasons, systemic (IV) stem cell therapy is the most advanced treatment. The treatments are safe, and they target the specific cause(s) of your problem. Stem cells for this therapy can be harvested from several sources:

- They can be aspirated from your bone marrow, usually in the hip area. They are then concentrated into a Bone Marrow Aspirate Concentrate (BMAC).

- They can also be taken from your adipose (fat) tissue through a mini liposuction. This is an outpatient procedure.

- Amniotic fluid from consenting donors is FDA regulated and contains a significant amount of growth factors and stem cell activators.

Whether from bone marrow, adipose tissue, or amniotic fluid, a potent stem cell solution is then prepared and injected. This solution is very concentrated; it contains a very large number of stem cells that can immediately go to work where they are needed, triggering the healing process without delay.

Systemic conditions that can be treated by IV stem cell therapy include diabetes, kidney failure, neurological conditions, and COPD, to name a few. Cardiac failure conditions may also be treated effectively with this type of therapy. I believe the future of the efficacy of IV stem cell injections is very promising.

TREATMENTS FOR VARIOUS CONDITIONS

There is no doubt that I am a true proponent of and highly recommend stem cell treatment/therapy because of what I, as well as thousands of other people, have experienced. But to broaden the scope of possible treatment options, it makes a lot of sense to me to expand your search to be pain-free.

There are never any guarantees when it comes to which procedure will work for you. But there is one guarantee I can attest to—if you do nothing, you will never know.

I created the following chart by choosing several musculoskeletal conditions that you may be struggling with now or think you may be on a path to be struggling with in the future. I included the symptoms and root causes to better inform you of what to look for so you can identify your condition, as well as several possible applications that are available to you.

You will also see a second chart of conventional medical procedures and natural alternative applications per condition. By having more knowledge about these specific areas—whether caused by injury, accident, illness, or the just plain old aging process—you will be better equipped to make the right decision for your health.

Keep in mind, there are never any guarantees when it comes to which procedure will work for you. But there is one guarantee I can attest to—if you do nothing, you will never know.

CHART 2.1: MUSCULOSKELETAL CONDITIONS AND SYMPTOMS, ROOT CAUSES, AND POSSIBLE APPLICATIONS/PROCEDURES

DEGENERATIVE DISC DISEASE

Degenerative disc disease (DDD) is referred to as arthritis of the back and occurs in many people during the normal aging process. As a person ages, the shock-absorbing pads, or discs, found between the vertebral bodies tend to collapse upon one another due to loss of elasticity. The nerve roots or spinal cord is compressed, causing local and radiating pain from the back down one or both legs.

SYMPTOMS
- Radiating pain traveling into legs and feet
- Pain worsens with long periods of standing or sitting
- Throbbing pain in lower back
- Stiffness in lower back

ROOT CAUSES
- Obesity; additional pressure on the joints, discs, nerves
- Heavy, repetitive lifting; improper lifting
- Injury, trauma
- Disc change, normal aging process
- Smoking

TREATMENT OPTIONS

Natural—Nonsurgical Procedures
- Stem cell therapy/treatment
- PRP (platelet-rich plasma) injections
- Regenerative orthopedic (prolotherapy) injections
- Adult stem cell activator/CNSN (section 2)
- Physical therapy, antigravity stretches

- Core exercises to enhance stability and support
- Chinese herbal medicine and herbal patches
- Food selection based on blood type
- Acupuncture
- Chiropractic care

Medical—Nonsurgical Procedures
- Spinal epidural, cortisone injections
- Medications

Medical—Surgical Procedures (only when all else fails)
- Surgical decompression—easing the pressure on the nerve roots, or spinal cord, by removing bone spurs and/ or portions of the lamina or enlarging the foramina
- Disc replacement—removing the dysfunctional disc and replacing it with an artificial prosthesis
- Posterolateral fusion—stabilizing the spine with screws and rods
- Anterior lumbar interbody fusion (ALIF)—surgically replacing the damaged disc with a spacer with bone graft; an advanced decompression surgery through the abdomen
- Posterior transforaminal interbody fusion—same as ALIF except the approach is through the back; pedicle screws are used to assist in the fusion of the vertebral joints

HERNIATED DISC

The rupture of a piece of a disc is referred to as a herniated disc. A herniated disc is sometimes referred to as a bulging or degenerative disc and causes pressure on the spinal cord or nerve.

SYMPTOMS
- Pain or stiffness in the back that makes it difficult to stand up straight or walk

- Radiating or traveling pain down one or both legs and/or arms causing numbness and/or weakness

ROOT CAUSE
- Collapsed disc
- Weak vertebral ligaments
- Poor posture, improper heavy lifting
- Accident or trauma

TREATMENT OPTIONS

Natural—Nonsurgical Procedures
- Physical therapy
- Stem cell therapy/treatment
- PRP (platelet-rich plasma) injections
- Regenerative orthopedic (prolotherapy) injections
- Adult stem cell activator/CNSN (section 2)
- Chinese herbal medicine and herbal patches
- Food selection based on blood type
- Acupuncture
- Chiropractic care

Medical—Nonsurgical Procedures
- Pain medications
- Spinal epidural, cortisone injections

Medical—Surgical Procedures (only when all else fails)
- Surgery

INFECTIONS/DISCITIS

Discitis is the inflammation of the vertebral disc space (discs and spinal bones).

SYMPTOMS

- Achy pain
- Fever
- Tenderness

ROOT CAUSES

- Blood infections or urine infections (urinary tract infections)

TREATMENT OPTIONS

Natural—Nonsurgical Procedures

- Adult stem cell activators (section 2)
- Chinese herbal medicine and herbal patches
- Food selection based on blood type

Medical—Nonsurgical Procedures

- Antibiotics

Medical—Surgical Procedures (only when all else fails)

- Possible surgery

OSTEOARTHRITIS

Osteoarthritis describes the changes that occur in joints as we age. Osteoarthritis is referred to as arthritis of the hips (spine), wear and tear arthritis, or degenerative joint disease. Over time, in the joints of hips or knees, which are weight-bearing joints, there is a wearing away of the cartilage, the protective material that prevents bone-on-bone friction. Some of the changes can be in the form of narrowing of the spinal joints, cysts, and bone spurs. Osteoarthritis in the lower back causes aches and stiffness.

SYMPTOMS

- Stiffness, pain, or aches in the lower back

ROOT CAUSES

- Fractures from traumas
- Aging

TREATMENT OPTIONS

Natural—Nonsurgical Procedures

- Stem cell therapy/treatment
- PRP (platelet-rich plasma) injections
- Regenerative orthopedic (prolotherapy) injections
- Adult stem cell activator/OST (section 2)
- Chinese herbal medicine and herbal patches
- Food selection based on blood type
- Physical therapy (PT)
- Dietary supplementation
- Acupuncture
- Apitherapy (bee venom therapy)
- Chiropractic care

Medical—Nonsurgical Procedures

- Medications

OSTEOPOROSIS OF THE SPINE

Osteoporosis of the spine is a painful degenerative condition that is a result of bone density loss. This condition causes bones to weaken, making them very susceptible to fractures from falls. Osteoporosis is common among the elderly and women, and occurs in the hips and spine.

SYMPTOMS

- Curvature of the spine
- Loss of normal height
- Pain brought on by fractured bone

ROOT CAUSES

- Menopause
- Aging process
- Falls or trauma
- Calcium and vitamin D deficiency
- Acidosis/pH imbalance
- Hormone imbalance

TREATMENT OPTIONS

Natural—Nonsurgical Procedures

- Stem cell therapy/treatment
- PRP (platelet-rich plasma) injections
- Regenerative orthopedic (prolotherapy) injections
- Adult stem cell activators/OST (section 2)
- Food selection based on blood type; balance pH
- Chinese herbal medicine and herbal patches
- Hormone replacement treatment (HRT)
- Nutritional supplements
- Acupuncture

Medical—Nonsurgical Procedures

- Medications

RHEUMATOID ARTHRITIS (RA)

Rheumatoid arthritis (RA) is an autoimmune disease where the body's immune system attacks its own joints and joint tissue. RA can cause inflammation of the joints and joint tissues. RA is characterized by flare-ups and remissions and can affect multiple joints or singular joints. When inflammation is chronic, the disease can cause joint destruction and deformity.

SYMPTOMS

The symptoms are painful swelling of the joints, stiffness, and joint dysfunction. Joint damage or degeneration can occur from RA.

ROOT CAUSE

RA is the result of an overactive immune system response.

TREATMENT OPTIONS

Natural—Nonsurgical Procedures

- Stem cell therapy/treatment
- PRP (platelet-rich plasma) injections
- Regenerative orthopedic (prolotherapy) injections
- Adult stem cell activator/CNT (section 2)
- Chinese herbal medicine and herbal patches
- Food selection based on blood type
- Apitherapy (bee venom therapy)
- Exercise—stretching, water exercises/aerobics
- Nutritional supplementation

Medical—Nonsurgical Procedures

- Medications

SCIATICA

Sciatica is nerve pain that travels from the spine down one or both legs below the knee(s) and into the feet. Sciatica causes numbness, tingling, and even weakness in the legs. It is referred to as either inflammation or compression of one or more of the branches of the sciatic nerve.

SYMPTOMS

- Searing or burning sensation

ROOT CAUSES

- Compression of piriformis or gluteus muscles of the buttocks, impinging on the branch nerve

- Occurs in the lower back (spine/discs) and/or sacrum deep into the gluteus muscles
- Impingement of bulging discs or narrowing of nerve canal/stenosis
- The sciatic nerve can be inflamed from continual impingement or pressure

TREATMENT OPTIONS

Natural—Nonsurgical Procedures
- Physical therapy, core exercises, stretching
- Stem cell/PRP (platelet-rich plasma) injections
- Regenerative orthopedic (prolotherapy) injections
- Adult stem cell activator/CNSN (section 2)
- Chinese herbal medicine and herbal patches
- Food selection based on blood type
- Acupuncture
- Chiropractic care

Medical—Nonsurgical Procedures
- Pain medications
- Spinal epidural, cortisone injections

Medical—Surgical Procedures (only when all else fails)
- Surgery

SPONDYLOLISTHESIS

The slippage of one vertebral body upon another due to arthritis, fracture, or trauma is referred to as spondylolisthesis.

SYMPTOMS

This condition can cause nerve pain due to slippage and spinal instability.

ROOT CAUSE

- Usually inherited at childhood or adolescence

TREATMENT OPTIONS

Natural—Nonsurgical Procedures

- Adult stem cell activator/CNSN (section 2)
- Physical therapy, core exercises
- Stem cell therapy/treatment
- PRP (platelet-rich plasma) injections
- Regenerative orthopedic (prolotherapy) injections
- Chinese herbal medicine and herbal patches
- Food selection based on blood type

Medical—Nonsurgical Procedures

- Pain medications
- Spinal epidural, cortisone injections

Medical—Surgical Procedures (only when all else fails)

- Surgery

STENOSIS (BACK)

Stenosis is a narrowing of the spinal canal or the foramen. This area or opening allows the nerve roots to pass through unrestricted. When degeneration occurs in the form of cysts, bone spurs, and even collapsed discs, the opening starts narrowing and causes pain and pressure on the nerve roots and spinal cord. This narrowing can occur anywhere in the spinal column.

SYMPTOMS

- Cervical spine (neck)—tightness in the neck; pain traveling down the arms into the fingers and hands; difficulty using hands; loss of strength due to pain, numbness

- Lumbar spine—lower body, buttocks, and legs feel heavy or weak; walking for long periods causes pain; numbness and weakness and cramping in the lower limbs

ROOT CAUSES

- Cervical spine (neck)—degenerative changes such as arthritic buildup or bone spurs that press against nerves; herniated discs can cause pressure on or compression of the nerves
- Lumbar spine—less spinal canal space for nerves to pass freely; necrosis or lack of blood flow

TREATMENT OPTIONS

Natural—Nonsurgical Procedures

- Physical therapy, antigravity stretches
- Stem cell therapy/treatment
- PRP (platelet-rich plasma) injections
- Regenerative orthopedic (prolotherapy) injections
- Adult stem cell activators/CNSN (section 2)
- Chinese herbal medicine and herbal patches
- Food selection based on blood type
- Acupuncture

Medical—Nonsurgical Procedures

- Spinal epidural, cortisone injections
- Pain and/or anti-inflammatory medications

Medical—Surgical Procedures (only when all else fails)

- Cervical laminectomy—removal of lamina and spinous process to relieve pressure, pain on spinal cord (neck)
- Surgical decompression—easing the pressure on the nerve roots or spinal cord by removing bone spurs and/or portions of the lamina or enlarging the foramina

- Posterolateral fusion—stabilizing the spine with screws and rods
- Anterior lumbar interbody fusion (ALIF)—surgically replacing the damaged disc with a spacer with bone graft; an advanced decompression surgery through the abdomen
- Posterior transforaminal interbody fusion—same as ALIF except approach is through the back; pedicle screws are used to assist in the fusion of the vertebral joints

CHART 2.2: INJURIES

BONE SPURS

Bone spurs are also referred to as osteophytes, which are projections of the body's normal bone structure. Common sites for bone spurs are the hips, knees, spine, hands, shoulders, and feet. When this calcification grows and touches or presses on other tissue or nerves, it can be very painful.

SYMPTOMS

- Numbness, pain, and tenderness
- Painful spots on the feet or heels when pressure from body weight is applied
- Some spurs, if located in a joint, can disrupt normal joint function

ROOT CAUSES

- Tendonitis, osteoarthritis, and even the aging process
- This can happen in the spine and feet
- The soft cartilage tissue that covers the ends of bones starts to break up, causing pain and swelling

TREATMENT OPTIONS

Natural—Nonsurgical Procedures
- Weight loss to lessen the pressure on the painful area
- Adult stem cell activator OST/OPTIWEIGHT (section 2)
- Ice therapy
- Rest
- Food selection based on blood type
- Supplement for lack of trace minerals (see appendix)

Medical—Nonsurgical Procedures
- Medications
- Cortisone injections

Medical—Surgical Procedures
- Surgery; see chart 2.1

CARPAL TUNNEL SYNDROME

Carpal tunnel is a narrow, rigid passageway of ligaments and bones at the base of the hand. It houses the median nerve and tendons that run down from the forearm. Carpal tunnel syndrome is when the median nerve gets pressed or squeezed at the wrist and becomes irritated and/or inflamed. This condition becomes very painful.

SYMPTOMS
- Gradual burning sensation
- Tingling and/or itching in palm of hand, fingers, thumb, index and middle fingers

ROOT CAUSES
- Trauma or injury to the wrist, swelling
- Sprain or fracture, swelling and pain
- Overactive pituitary gland
- Water retention during pregnancy

- Joint stress
- RA

TREATMENT OPTIONS

Natural—Nonsurgical Procedures
- Rest, immobilize the wrist
- Ice packs
- Natural diuretics, vitamin B_6
- Stem cell therapy/treatment
- PRP (platelet-rich plasma) injections
- Regenerative orthopedic (prolotherapy) injections
- Adult stem cell activator/CNSN (section 2)
- Chinese herbal medicine and herbal patches

Medical—Nonsurgical Procedures
- Nonsteroidal anti-inflammatory drugs (NSAIDs)
- Medication, anti-inflammatory
- Orally administered diuretics
- Corticosteroid injections

Medical—Surgical Procedures (only when all else fails)
- Surgery

FRACTURES (SPINE)

Fractures are spinal bones that are not completely cracked through such as a break. They are usually surface cracks that can occur due to a fall, accident, or trauma. They are common in osteoporosis patients who experience minimal traumas or falls.

SYMPTOMS

- Pain
- Instability of balance

ROOT CAUSES

- Falls
- Trauma
- Accidents

TREATMENT OPTIONS

Natural—Nonsurgical Procedures

- Physical therapy
- Stem cell therapy/treatment
- PRP (platelet-rich plasma) injections
- Regenerative orthopedic (prolotherapy) injections
- Adult stem cell activator/OST (section 2)
- Chinese herbal medicine and herbal patches
- Rest and use of bracing
- Food selection based on blood type

Medical—Nonsurgical Procedures

- Pain medications
- Spinal epidural, cortisone injections

Medical—Surgical Procedures (only when all else fails)

- Bone grafting

HIPS

Hip pain is a common problem and can be confusing as there are several causes. It is important to have an accurate diagnosis of the cause of your symptoms (not just the symptoms) so the appropriate modality or treatment can be directed at the root cause. The hip joints are more complicated than other joints and therefore should have a thorough examination—including examination of the soft tissue or connective tissue that supports the joint—before determining what treatment is necessary.

SYMPTOMS

- Sharp pain
- Burning pain
- Pain on the outside of the hip joint (greater trochanter)
- Pain on the inside of the hip joint (groin)
- Difficulty walking
- Aggravated by prolonged sitting and standing

ROOT CAUSES

- Arthritis—This is the most common and frequent cause of hip pain. There are many natural treatments available. If all else fails, then hip replacement may be your only option.
- Trochanteric bursitis—A very common condition that causes inflammation of the bursa over the outside of the hip joint.
- Tendonitis—This can happen in any of the tendons that attach to the hip joint. The most common area where tendonitis occurs is around the hip, where the iliotibial band (IT band) attaches. It is commonly referred to as iliotibial band tendonitis.
- Osteonecrosis—This is a condition that occurs when the blood flow to an area of a bone is disrupted or restricted. Without sufficient blood flow, the cells die off and the bone can collapse. This is common in someone with hip pain.
- Referred pain, lumbar pain—Pain that is felt in the buttocks and hips can often come from the spinal cord. This usually means a disc is herniated and/or sciatic nerve impingement.
- Snapping hip syndrome—This condition causes a loud snapping sound and can occur in three areas: 1) where the IT band snaps over the outside of the thigh; 2) where torn cartilage of the hip socket and/or labrum causes a snapping feeling; and 3) where the hip flexor snaps over the front of the hip joint.

- Muscle strains—Strained hamstring muscles or groin pulls can cause hip pain, while surrounding strained muscles and muscle spasms of the hip can contribute to hip pain.
- Hip fractures—Osteoporosis patients and the elderly can experience hip fractures. Surgical procedures are required to mend this condition.
- Stress fractures—Participation in high-impact sports is a common cause of stress fractures.
- Pelvis ligaments and tendons—Improperly healed ligaments or ligaments that have been overstretched cannot properly support the hip joint, causing intense joint pain. Tendons that may be torn at the bone will cause lack of support for the hip joint, causing intense pain as well.

TREATMENT OPTIONS

Natural—Nonsurgical Procedures
- Stem cell therapy/treatment
- PRP (platelet-rich plasma) injections
- Regenerative orthopedic (prolotherapy) injections
- Adult stem cell activator/OST (section 2)
- Chinese herbal medicine and herbal patches
- Rest
- Ice and heat therapy
- Ultrasound
- Chiropractic care

Medical—Nonsurgical Procedures
- Nonsteroidal anti-inflammatory drugs (NSAIDs)
- Pain and anti-inflammatory medications

Medical—Surgical Procedures
- Total hip replacement
- Partial hip replacement

LATERAL EPICONDYLITIS (TENNIS ELBOW)

The inflammation of the tendons of the elbow, usually those on the outer side of the elbow joint, is referred to as lateral epicondylitis.

SYMPTOMS
- Severe pain radiating from elbow into the forearm and wrist

ROOT CAUSES
- Poor sports technique: tennis, golf
- Repetitive use: commercial painters, construction workers (such as plumbers)
- Excessive use: culinary motions like continually cutting veggies and meats

TREATMENT OPTIONS

Natural—Nonsurgical Procedures
- Stem cell therapy/treatment
- PRP (platelet-rich plasma) injections
- Regenerative orthopedic (prolotherapy) injections
- Adult stem cell activator/CNT (section 2)
- Exercise
- Rest
- Physical therapy
- Chinese herbal medicine and herbal patches

Medical—Nonsurgical Procedures
- Nonsteroidal anti-inflammatory drugs (NSAIDs)

Medical—Surgical Procedures (only when all else fails)
- Surgery

MUSCLE SPASM/MUSCLE CRAMP

Muscle spasms, charley horses, or muscle cramps, as they are called, can happen at any time unexpectedly. The muscle spasm is when the muscle in the calf, thigh, foot, or arm suddenly becomes rock hard and very tight.

SYMPTOMS

- Extreme pain
- Very tight muscle

ROOT CAUSES

- Dehydration
- Poor blood circulation
- Muscle fatigue; exercising in the heat
- Nutrient deficiency (magnesium, potassium, and calcium)
- Insufficient stretching and overexertion of the calf muscle
- Side effects from medications

TREATMENT OPTIONS

Natural—Nonsurgical Procedures

- Massaging and stretching the muscle
- Icing the muscle or warming the muscle; Epsom salt bath or Jacuzzi

Medical—Nonsurgical Procedures

- None

Note: If you frequently experience cramps or spasms for no apparent reason, you should speak to your doctor, as they could signal a medical problem that requires treatment.

ROTATOR CUFF INJURY

When the tendons of the shoulder joint (ball and socket) area are painfully inflamed, irritated, and swollen, this condition is referred to as rotator cuff tendonitis (RCT). RCT affects men and women of all ages.

SYMPTOMS

- Pain when moving the shoulder upward, outward, or across the body
- Pain when sleeping or lying on bad shoulder, difficulty pulling the covers over the body
- All overhead lifting or working that requires raising the shoulders is painful

ROOT CAUSES

- Many sports activities with repetitive movements: overhead rotation, pitching motion in baseball, lifting and/or pressing weights overhead, swimming
- Career/hobby: golf swing, construction worker, painter
- Chronic inflammation (months) can induce tears of the tendon tissue
- Age-related: forty-plus group, weekend warriors repetitiously throwing football, baseball

TREATMENT OPTIONS

Natural—Nonsurgical Procedures
- Chinese herbal medicine and herbal patches
- Stem cell therapy/treatment
- PRP (platelet-rich plasma) injections
- Regenerative orthopedic (prolotherapy) injections
- Adult stem cell activator/CNT (section 2)
- Applying ice pack to shoulder
- Physical therapy
- Chiropractic care

- Rest
- Avoiding activities that irritate the shoulders

Medical—Nonsurgical Procedures
- Nonsteroidal anti-inflammatory drugs
- Cortisone steroid injections

Medical Surgical Procedures (only when all else fails)
- Surgery

SPRAIN

A sprain is a stretch and/or tear of a ligament, the fibrous band of connective tissue that joins the end of one bone with another. Ligaments stabilize and support the body's joints. There are three levels of sprain severity:

- A severe sprain causes excruciating pain at the moment of injury. This is when the ligament tears completely from the bone, causing the joint to become nonfunctional.
- A moderate sprain produces a partial tear of the ligament. This condition contributes to instability and swelling of the joint.
- A mild sprain causes a stretched ligament, but the joint remains stabilized.

SYMPTOMS

Inflammation, pain, bruising, swelling, and inflammation are common to all three categories of sprains: mild, moderate, severe. The individual will usually feel a tear or pop in the joint.

ROOT CAUSES

A sprain is caused directly or indirectly by a fall or hit to the body, or a trauma. The trauma can be such that it knocks a joint out of position, overstretches the supporting ligaments, and in severe cases ruptures the supporting ligaments. Typically this injury occurs when an individual turns the ankle while playing sports, running, or stepping on an uneven surface, or maybe lands wrong on an outstretched arm. Anybody is susceptible to a sprain, from athletes to people who are overweight and in poor condition.

TREATMENTS OPTIONS

Natural—Nonsurgical Procedures
- Stem cell therapy/treatment
- PRP (platelet-rich plasma) injections
- Regenerative orthopedic (prolotherapy) injections
- Adult stem cell activator/CNT (section 2)
- Rest, ice, compression, and elevation (RICE)

Medical—Nonsurgical Procedures
- Mild condition—medical doctor evaluation of the injury to establish treatment and rehabilitation plan
- Severe sprain—may require surgery or immobilization followed by months of therapy

STRAIN

A strain is an injury of a muscle and/or tendon. Tendons are fibrous cords of tissue that attach muscles to bone. There are three levels or stages of strain:
- Severe strain—partial or full rupture of a muscle and/or tendon; this leaves the individual incapacitated. Acute strains are caused by a direct hit to the body, over-stretching, or excessive muscle contraction.
- Moderate strain—loss of some muscle function where the torn muscle/tendon has been overstretched
- Mild strain—a slight muscle/tendon stretched or pulled

SYMPTOMS
- Pain
- Muscle spasms and weakness
- Swelling

- Inflammation
- Cramping

ROOT CAUSES

Chronic strains are the result of overuse (prolonged, repetitive movement) of muscles and tendons. Inadequate rest breaks during intensive training precipitates a strain. Anybody is susceptible to a strain, from athletes to people who are overweight and in poor condition.

TREATMENT OPTIONS

Natural—Nonsurgical Procedures
- Stem cell therapy/treatment
- PRP (platelet-rich plasma) injections
- Regenerative orthopedic (prolotherapy) injections
- Adult stem cell activator/CNT (section 2)
- Rest, ice, compression, and elevation (RICE)

Medical—Nonsurgical Procedures
- Mild strain—medical doctor evaluation of the injury to establish treatment and rehabilitation plan
- Severe strain—may require surgery or immobilization followed by months of therapy

Note: To reduce your risk of injury:
- Exercise to build muscle strength
- Stretch daily
- Wear properly fitting shoes
- Eat for your blood type
- Warm up before sports or recreational activities

TENDONITIS

Irritation or inflammation of a tendon is referred to as tendonitis. This condition affects any one of the fibrous cords that attach the bone to muscle. Tendonitis can occur in any joint of the body but usually occurs in the shoulders, elbows, wrists, ankles, and hips. Overuse or repetitive use is generally the cause in many types of sports: tennis (elbow), swimming (shoulders), golf (elbow), baseball (pitchers' shoulders), even track and field (jumpers' knees).

SYMPTOMS (AT THE ATTACHMENT OF THE TENDON AT THE BONE)
- Dull pain
- Tenderness
- Mild swelling

ROOT CAUSES
- Overuse; repetitive use over time
- Explosive injury, extreme force of the joint
- Irritation of a weakened tendon

TREATMENT

Natural—Nonsurgical Procedures
- Stem cell therapy/treatment
- PRP (platelet-rich plasma) injections
- Regenerative orthopedic (prolotherapy) injections
- Adult stem cell activator/CNT (section 2)
- Chinese herbal medicine and herbal patches
- Rest and ice
- Food selection based on blood type
- Exercises; stretches and strengthening joint and surrounding muscles

Medical—Nonsurgical Procedures
- Nonsteroidal anti-inflammatory drugs (NSAIDs)
- Corticosteroid injections to reduce inflammation (Note: These injections can be damaging to the tendon, with repeated injections potentially weakening it and leading to a tendon rupture.)

TENDON TEAR

Tendons are fibrous tissue that attaches bone to muscle. An injury to the tendon is referred to as a strain or tear, and rehabilitation is dependent upon the severity of the injury or tear. Tendons, in rare circumstances, can rupture or snap, but can handle forces upward to five times a person's body weight. Injuries to tendons are classified on a sliding scale of first-, second-, and third-degree strains. Tendon injuries are common for people with an O blood type.

SYMPTOMS

- First-degree strain—pain and discomfort; easiest to heal or rehabilitate
- Second-degree strain—major pain, discoloration, and swelling
- Third-degree strain—complete tear, joint instability, and muscle dysfunction

ROOT CAUSES

Injuries to tendons usually occur when involving joints that move in more than one direction: ankles, wrists, shoulders, and hips.

TREATMENT OPTIONS

Natural—Nonsurgical Procedures

- First-degree strain—rest, ice, compression, and elevation (RICE)
- Second-degree strain—RICE
- Stem cell therapy/treatment
- PRP (platelet-rich plasma) injections
- Regenerative orthopedic (prolotherapy) injections
- Adult stem cell activator/CNT (section 2)
- Chinese herbal medicine and herbal patches
- Food selection based on blood type

Medical—Nonsurgical Procedures
- Second-degree strain—anti-inflammatory medications, analgesics, RICE

Medical—Surgical Procedures (only when all else fails)
- Third-degree strain—surgical repair; lengthy rehabilitation

Note: Thorough stretching and strengthening of surrounding muscles to increase the range of motion (ROM) of a joint will prevent possible tendon injury.

TORN LIGAMENTS

Ligaments are dense fibrous connective tissue comprised of attenuated collagenous fibers. They are viscoelastic and can be stretched but only to a limit as they can tear when overstretched. Joints are stabilized and strengthened by ligaments. Ligaments connect bone to bone. Ligaments stabilize the joint and the articular capsule. An untreated ligament tear will lead to joint instability and eventually lead to cartilage wear and possibly osteoarthritis.

SYMPTOMS
- Snapping or cracking sound
- Pain
- Painful bruising and swelling

ROOT CAUSES
- Overstretching
- Hyperlaxity, double-jointedness = overstretching the ligament

TREATMENT OPTIONS

Natural—Nonsurgical Procedures
- Stem cell therapy/treatment
- PRP (platelet-rich plasma) injections

- Regenerative orthopedic (prolotherapy) injections
- Adult stem cell activator/CNT (section 2)
- Chinese herbal medicine and herbal patches

Medical—Surgical Procedures (only when all else fails)
- Surgery

TORN MENISCUS (KNEE)

Torn meniscus is when the C-shaped pieces of cartilage around the knee are injured. The actual cartilage tissue that is very fibrous becomes frayed like a rope that starts tearing apart. This condition can be extremely painful, causing temporary disability and dysfunctional movement at the knee joint, particularly because it is a weight-bearing joint.

SYMPTOMS
- Pain when turning or twisting
- Stiffness
- Swelling
- Popping sounds due to swollen tissue
- Difficulty straightening the knee

ROOT CAUSES
- Sudden twisting or exertion or start-and-stop motions
- Long periods of kneeling, squatting, or poor position when lifting
- Athletics: torn meniscus can accompany an anterior cruciate ligament injury, causing tremendous swelling, inflammation, and pain

TREATMENT OPTIONS

Natural—Nonsurgical Procedures
- Rest; avoid any activity or movement that would irritate the knee joint

- Ice; reduces swollen tissue and reduces pain (inflammation = pain)
- Stem cell therapy/treatment
- PRP (platelet-rich plasma) injections
- Regenerative orthopedic (prolotherapy) injections
- Adult stem cell activator/CNT (section 2)
- Chinese herbal medical and herbal patches
- Exercise: physical therapy to strengthen surrounding muscles of the knee to stabilize the knee joint

Medical—Nonsurgical Procedures
- Medication: Nonsteroidal anti-inflammatory drugs reduce inflammation and ease pain
- Orthotics: arch support for balanced weight distribution

Medical—Surgical Procedures (only after all else fails)
- Surgery

WHIPLASH

This is a soft tissue injury to the muscles and ligaments in the back of the neck.

SYMPTOMS
- Severe pain
- Muscle spasms
- Stiffness in the back of the neck

ROOT CAUSES
- Most often caused by a rear-end motor vehicle collision
- A sudden hyperextension movement (head being whipped backward) followed by hyperflexion of the neck (head being whipped forward)

TREATMENT OPTIONS

Natural—Nonsurgical Procedures

- Soft foam cervical collar (for stability)
- Physical therapy exercises for reducing pain and stiffness and regaining function
- Chinese herbal medicine and herbal patches
- Acupuncture
- Stem cell therapy/treatment
- PRP (platelet-rich plasma) injections
- Regenerative orthopedic (prolotherapy) injections
- Adult stem cell activator/CNT (section 2)
- Chiropractic care

Medical—Nonsurgical Procedures

- Nonsteroidal anti-inflammatory drugs

After taking a closer look at some common injuries and musculoskeletal conditions along with the various treatments/therapies and possible applications, I hope you will be able to make a wiser and more accurate decision for treatment should you become prey to any of them. Injuries don't happen to just you and me. Let's see how world-class professional athletes address their sports injuries.

STEM CELL THERAPY FOR SPORT INJURIES

We all tend to look up to our favorite sports figures. We watch them perform and cheer them on as they win championships or titles. Some of us even follow how they eat and how they train. But what about the way they treat their injuries? Let's face it, they have much more to lose (financially) from an injury than you or I!

What have professional sports figures like Tiger Woods (PGA), Kobe Bryant (NBA), Peyton Manning (NFL), Dwight Howard (NBA), Fred Couples (PGA), Bartolo Colon (MLB), and others done for their sports injuries? They've turned to stem cell therapy.

There are many types of sports injuries, and they can involve almost any area of the body. Here are some common types.

BASIC SPORTS INJURY TYPES/CATEGORIES

1. Bone injuries—breaks, fractures, and "bruising"

2. Soft tissue injuries—muscles, ligaments, tendons, cartilage, and skin scrapes and bruises

3. Joint injuries—dislocations, separations, and post-injury arthritis

4. Overuse injuries—damage to ligaments/tendons or joints caused by repetitive activities

5. Head injuries—primarily concussions

The specific areas of injury include muscle, bone, joint, head, and overuse injuries. Stem cell treatments/therapies are used to speed the healing process and enhance recovery to lessen the amount of down time. The sooner the injuries are repaired, the sooner the athlete can return to the playing field.

Stem cell treatments/therapies are used to promote recovery in areas that historically heal poorly or not at all. These include tendon and ligament injuries, cartilage injuries, repeated concussions, and some overuse and muscle injuries.

As you've learned thus far, stem cells are unique cells in our bodies. Because of the ease with which stem cells can be taken from adipose tissue (body fat) and its abundance of stem cells, sports physicians use fat-derived adult stem cells from the athlete to treat sports injuries.

We also learned that adult stem cells have a couple of unique genetic characteristics. Let's see how they apply in the sports arena.

1. Replication/self-renewal
Adult stem cells can replicate or multiply themselves. Once injected into an injured or damaged area(s), the stem cells will multiply in number. This replication factor enhances their ability to aid in rapid healing and recovery.

2. Differentiation
Stem cells can turn into, or become, other types of cells. Using "fat-derived" stem cells, the adult stem cells are converted into new cell types such as cartilage, muscle, skin, and bone cells.

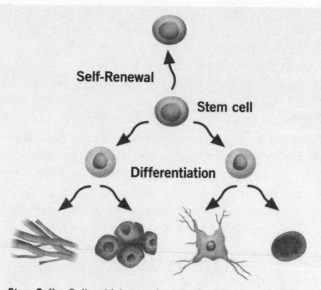

Stem Cells: Cells which are characterized by their ability to renew themselves through cell division. They also possess the ability to develop into other cell types (differentiation).

Unlike conventional medicine, the use of adult stem cells and their unique genetic characteristics for the treatment of sports injuries (and similar injuries outside of sports) can result in much more rapid repair and healing of the injuries. This shortens the time of recovery and allows the athlete to return to his or her sport. These are other reasons why stem cell therapy is so disruptive.

OK, so you are not a professional athlete, but you do participate in recreational sports. You enjoy playing tennis with your tennis team, but now your elbow is terribly painful. Or your knees are starting to kill you. Or you can't walk around the house very well because your heels are so painful from those long runs you have been taking every day.

THE BANDAGE SYNDROME

Unfortunately, your favorite sports and activities that used to thrill you are now becoming more problematic than fun. Now you are dealing with the pain and discomfort from your sports injury, which is carrying over into your everyday life.

Thus far, you've found some relief from ice and heat treatments, had a couple of massages, used topical oils and creams, and exhausted the over-the-counter medications (NSAIDs) until your liver is screaming for some relief. The only thing left is to take time off from your sport or recreational activity.

What can you and millions like you do? Are there any other options available for healing and repairing your injuries, other than using those bandages that only mask the symptoms?

The great news is that anyone can take advantage of stem cell therapy or PRP therapy just like the professionals do. These disruptive treatments/therapies are proven, safe, effective, and less expensive alternatives to dangerous and costly orthopedic joint, tendon, and spine surgeries.

The conventional medicine mind-set approach to fixing injuries by performing surgeries is a thing of the past. Today, stem cell therapy and PRP therapy are becoming the norm in regenerative medicine.

FREQUENTLY ASKED QUESTIONS

Who is a candidate for stem cell therapy?

Almost everyone! Although some people have such extreme damage that stem cells may not be an answer, I encourage everyone to at least look into it. In the past, if a patient had serious joint dysfunction or persistent musculoskeletal pain in the knee, back, shoulder, elbow, hips, neck, or wrists, their options were very limited. The typical protocol choices were pain medication, steroid shots, and anti-inflammatories, then wait and see how you do. Lastly, the patient would face joint replacement surgery and hope it was successful.

Today you have another choice! Many scientists and doctors agree that stem cells are the medicine of the future. As far as orthopedic problems go, this approach is now available, and for many it may very well be the treatment of choice and yield a far superior result than more conventional approaches.

What does the treatment involve, and how does it work?

The procedure is nonsurgical and performed in an outpatient environment. Approximately 60–100 ccs (more in some cases) are harvested from a patient's own belly fat. After numbing the skin, this mini lipo-suction procedure is done with large syringes under low pressure and takes about forty-five minutes.

The stem cells are isolated through a special process in a lab that takes about ninety minutes. Then the isolated stem cells with growth factors are mixed with a simple blood draw (called platelet-rich plasma, or PRP). Next the stem cell/PRP combo is injected at the specific joint and ligament sites that are the root cause of the problem. The stem cells will remain alive for about six months, continuing to regenerate and multiply and rebuild the damaged tissues during that period. Within two to four hours the patient can go home.

What type of conditions can stem cell therapy treat?

Our findings are that stem cells have the capacity to regenerate all types of tissue, which includes cartilage, bone, ligaments, and tendons. Stem cells detect specific damaged tissues and then repair them selectively. Some conditions that can be treated include multiple sclerosis (MS), Parkinson's disease, rheumatoid arthritis, osteoarthritis, and chronic obstructive pulmonary disease (COPD).

Can stem cells from adipose tissue differentiate into cells other than fat, bone, and cartilage?

Several studies (1–9) have demonstrated that stem cells derived from adipose tissue can create a vast array of cell types, including neurons, which are potentially critical for treating many kinds of neurological diseases.

1. Kristine M. Safford et al. "Neurogenic Differentiation of Murine and Human Adipose-Derived Stromal Cells." *Biochemical and Biophysical Research Communications* 294, no. 2 (June 7, 2002): 371–379. https://doi.org/10.1016/S0006-291X(02)00469-2.

2. Peter H. Ashjian et al. "In Vitro Differentiation of Human Processed Lipoaspirate Cells Into Early Neural Progenitors." *Plastic and Reconstructive Surgery* (May 2003). 10.1097/01.PRS.0000055043.62589.05. https://doi.org/.

3. Soo Kyung Kang et al. "Neurogenesis of Rhesus Adipose Stromal Cells." *Journal of Cell Science* 117 (2004): 4289–4299. 10.1242/jcs.01264. https://doi.org/.

4. Min Jeong Seo et al. "Differentiation of Human Adipose Stromal Cells Into Hepatic Lineage In Vitro and In Vivo." *Biochemical and Biophysical Research*

Communications 328, no. 1 (March 4, 2005): 258–264. https://doi.org/10.1016/j.bbrc.2004.12.158.

5. Martin Brzoska et al. "Epithelial Differentiation of Human Adipose Tissue-Derived Adult Stem Cells." *Biochemical and Biophysical Research Communications* 330, no. 1 (April 29, 2005): 142–150. https://doi.org/10.1016/j.bbrc.2005.02.141.

6. Katharina Timper et al. "Human Adipose Tissue-Derived Mesenchymal Stem Cells Differentiate Into Insulin, Somatostatin, and Glucagon Expressing Cells." *Biochemical and Biophysical Research Communications* 341, no. 4 (March 24, 2006): 1135–1140. https://doi.org/10.1016/j.bbrc.2006.01.072.

7. Larissa V. Rodriguez et al. "Clonogenic Multipotent Stem Cells in Human Adipose Tissue Differentiate Into Functional Smooth Muscle Cells." *Proceedings of the National Academy of Sciences of the United States of America* 103, no. 32 (August 8, 2006): 12167–12172. https://dx.doi.org/10.1073%2Fpnas.0604850103.

8. S. Heydarkhan-Hagvall et al. "Human Adipose Stem Cells: A Potential Cell Source for Cardiovascular Tissue Engineering." *Cells Tissues Organs* 187 (2008): 263–274. https://doi.org/10.1159/000113407.

9. Yong Zhao et al. "Neurogenic Differentiation From Adipose-Derived Stem Cells and Application for Autologous Transplantation in Spinal Cord Injury." *Cell and Tissue Banking* 16, no. 3 (September 2015): 335–342. https://doi.org/10.1007/s10561-014-9476-3.

Can a person with Parkinson's disease benefit from stem cell therapy?

Two recent studies demonstrated that even unmanipulated mesenchymal stem cells reduced many of the symptoms experienced by individuals with Parkinson's disease (1–2). Additionally, the cellular mechanisms behind this therapeutic benefit have been extensively researched in an experimental setting (3–5).

1. N. K. Venkataramana et al. "Bilateral Transplantation of Allogenic Adult Human Bone Marrow-Derived Mesenchymal Stem Cells Into the Subventricular Zone of Parkinson's Disease: A Pilot Clinical Study." *Stem Cells International* 2012 (2012): 931902. https://dx.doi.org/10.1155%2F2012%2F931902.

2. N. K. Venkataramana et al. "Open-Labeled Study of Unilateral Autologous Bone-Marrow-Derived Mesenchymal Stem Cell Transplantation in Parkinson's Disease." *Translational Research* 155, no. 2 (February 2010): 62–70. http://dx.doi.org/10.1016/j.trsl.2009.07.006.

3. Lidia Cova et al. "Multiple Neurogenic and Neurorescue Effects of Human Mesenchymal Stem Cell After Transplantation in an Experimental Model of Parkinson's Disease." *Brain Research* 1311 (January 22, 2010): 12–27. https://doi.org/10.1016/j.brainres.2009.11.041.

4. Hyun Jung Park et al. "Mesenchymal Stem Cells Therapy Exerts Neuroprotection in a Progressive Animal Model of Parkinson's Disease." *Journal of Neurochemistry* 107, no. 1 (October 2008): 141–151. http://dx.doi.org/10.1111/j.1471-4159.2008.05589.x.

5. Yin Xia Chao et al. "Mesenchymal Stem Cell Transplantation Attenuates Blood Brain Barrier Damage and Neuroinflammation and Protects Dopaminergic Neurons Against MPTP Toxicity in the Substantia Nigra in a Model of Parkinson's Disease." *Journal of Neuroimmunology* 216, no. 1–2 (November 30, 2009): 39–50. http://dx.doi.org/10.1016/j.jneuroim.2009.09.003.

What other medical conditions may benefit from stem cell treatment?

In addition to the articles already cited, there is a growing body of medical literature demonstrating the potential benefits of stem cell therapy for many conditions ranging from musculoskeletal issues, such as osteoarthritis, to neurological issues, such as MS (1–6).

1. Anil Bhansali et al. "Efficacy and Safety of Autologous Bone Marrow-Derived Stem Cell Transplantation in Patients With Type 2 Diabetes Mellitus: A Randomized Placebo-Controlled Study." *Cell Transplantation* 23, no. 9 (2014): 1075–1085. https://doi.org/10.3727 /096368913X665576.

2. Peter Connick et al. "Autologous Mesenchymal Stem Cells for the Treatment of Secondary Progressive Multiple Sclerosis: An Open-Label Phase 2a Proof-Of-Concept Study." *Lancet Neurology* 11, no. 2 (February 2012): 150–156. https://dx.doi.org/10.1016 %2FS1474-4422(11)70305-2.

3. Ashu Bhasin et al. "Autologous Mesenchymal Stem Cells in Chronic Stroke." *Cerebrovascular Diseases Extra* 1, no. 1 (January–December 2011): 93–104. https://dx.doi .org/10.1159%2F000333381.

4. Osamu Honmou et al. "Intravenous Administration of Auto Serum-Expanded Autologous Mesenchymal Stem Cells in Stroke." *Brain* 134, no. 6 (June 2011): 1790–1807. https://dx.doi.org/10.1093%2Fbrain%2Fawr063.

5. Oh Young Bang et al. "Autologous Mesenchymal Stem Cell Transplantation in Stroke Patients." *Annals of Neurology* 57, no. 6 (June 2005): 874–882. http://dx.doi .org/10.1002/ana.20501.

6. Jin Soo Lee et al. "A Long-Term Follow-Up Study of Intravenous Autologous Mesenchymal Stem Cell Transplantation in Patients With Ischemic Stroke." *Stem Cells* 28, no. 6 (June 2010): 1099–1106. http://dx.doi.org /10.1002/stem.430.

Is stem cell therapy safe?

Orthopedic stem cell therapy is a minimally invasive and very safe procedure. The patient experiences only minimal soreness after their mini liposuction and the injections. There is no risk of infection, as the stem cells are those of the patient. Common sense, engaging in activities without weight bearing loads, plus stretching for the first few weeks are helpful for stem cell regeneration and tissue repair.

Can people with diabetes type 1 and diabetes type 2 be helped with stem cell therapy?

The use of adult adipose stem cell therapy as a new alternative treatment to help manage the complications of people with diabetes type 1 and diabetes type 2 is under way. The stem cells extracted from a patient may have the potential to replace countless cells of the body, insulin-producing cells included. The undifferentiated cells may heal the body by replacing cells plagued with disease by regenerating new cells.

What is the success rate?

While success rates vary widely among different conditions, there are promising results using adult stem cells for heart tissue regeneration, corneal reconstruction, treatment of spinal cord injuries, and treatment of autoimmune diseases such as diabetes and lupus. For example, a study of twenty-eight heart attack patients showed an average improvement of 4.8 percent in the heart's ability to pump blood after adult stem cell treatments an average of 4.7 days after their heart attacks. In a study of twenty patients who received corneal adult stem cell transplants, sixteen had improved vision. A clinical study of nineteen patients with auto-immune disorders, including lupus, revealed that 90 percent improved or experienced remission after being treated with their own stem cells.[1]

Some conditions show a higher rate of success with stem cell therapy, whereas other types of conditions have a lower rate of success. As more and more physicians improve their ability to effectively use stem cell therapy to treat various conditions via experience and repetition over time, rates of success will increase.

How does stem cell therapy help with osteoarthritis?

Generally, osteoarthritic patients must deal with cartilage deterioration at the end of their bones in the joints. This slippery tissue serves as a cushion that prevents friction or rubbing during motion. Over time, the cartilage wears down and the patient suffers from inflammation and pain due to the bones rubbing against each other. Once injected into the joint, the MSCs (mesenchymal stem cells) help reduce the inflammation and differentiate, or change, into new cartilage, or what is referred to as chondrocyte cells.

How long before the patient improves?

Patients often ask how long it will be before they feel improvement. Stem cells rely on a patient's own healing response, so it is impossible to predict who will heal more quickly. In some patients and some joints, the stem cells will ignite quickly and heal rapidly, and the patient may notice marked improvements even within the first week. For others, it may be six weeks before they experience improvement.

Is there a follow-up?

For those who have a very chronic condition, a four- to six-week PRP follow-up treatment may be most beneficial.

How long do the results last?

When stem cell therapy is a success and the joint or connective tissue structure is regenerated, there is every reason to believe that this will be a long-term solution. Keep in mind, with all patients being different and the severity of the condition varying, individual results will vary.

How many treatments does the patient need?

Depending on the tissue damage, severity of the condition, size of the area that needs to be injected, and most importantly, the patient's healing capability, people usually need a series of one to six treatments to improve. Each treatment is independent of all the others, meaning each treatment has benefits on its own.

How long is recovery time?

For most people, there is no downtime, and almost immediately to within twenty-four hours, pain relief is experienced. This makes it quite easy and comfortable for people to go back to work or assume their usual activities immediately.

How much does stem cell therapy cost?

Stem cell therapy is pricey, and the cost will vary among physicians. A blood draw plus the mini liposuction procedure, lab fees, and injections could range from $1,200 to $7,000 per site for a knee or shoulder joint. For a more complex joint, such as the lumbar spine or hip, or for multiple sites, the costs can be as high as $8,000 plus. Some physicians may discount the second or third sites by 50 percent. Many patients have two areas that require attention; in this case, the second area may be discounted 50 percent. If the patient cannot afford stem cell therapy, he or she can still benefit from PRP therapy. Though it would take several additional sessions, there is still hope for tissue repair and healing.

Is stem cell therapy covered by insurance?

There is high expectation that insurance companies will be covering this technology in the near future. Some stem cell clinics offer payment plans.

Why do most people seek out stem cell therapy?

It depends upon the individual, but most people have tried conventional medicine and practices and were not satisfied with the results. Some want to be pain-free, some are looking for increased range of motion, some need more strength, and some want to go back to activities they enjoy, like participating in their favorite sports. For others, it is important not to have to think twice about getting up only to get a glass of water, or just being able to walk again. In general, people who seek out stem cell therapy want to be functional again and enjoy an optimum quality of life.

Hopefully you have learned just a little more about stem cells in this section than you knew before. From the looks of the history and advancement of stem cell therapy over the years to today's widely expanded current treatments and therapies and new discoveries, its track record clearly has proven to be very promising. As stem cell therapy and treatments continue their course, it won't be too long before they will become the gold standard in regenerative and orthopedic medicine for people from all walks of life all over the world, far into the future.

As one who has experienced living with the debilitating condition of chronic pain and the awesome results I experienced (and still do) from stem cell treatments, I can't help but be an advocate of and believer in the hope the efficacious results stem cell therapy/treatments deliver.

If you are suffering with chronic joint pain, musculoskeletal injuries, neuropathy, degenerative diseases, or any of the other health conditions I've mentioned, I want to encourage you to seek out a physician who specializes in stem cell therapy. Don't live another day in pain and discomfort. Be willing to step out of the box of conventional medicine and embrace with confidence the hope of improved health and optimum life that stem cell therapy can offer you.

Should you need assistance in locating a stem cell physician, please feel free to call my office at 1-800-259-2639. To select a stem cell physician in your area, go to my website, www.stemcelldocs.net.

CHAPTER 3

PRP—A DISRUPTIVE THERAPY

I N THIS CHAPTER, I will reveal to you both my personal experiences and those of the medical field to illustrate how PRP therapy has surpassed the conventional medical procedures and has become the answer to many musculoskeletal conditions and more.

WHAT IS PRP THERAPY?

PRP (platelet-rich plasma), in my estimation, is another disruptive therapy and is somewhat like stem cell therapy. PRP therapy is an outpatient, nonsurgical procedure using small, precise injections of PRP—with or without stem cells—to regenerate damaged joints, ligaments, and tendons. The PRP is rich in your body's own growth factors and is spun down in a centrifuge from a simple blood draw in a process that takes about thirty minutes. (By contrast, as I explained in chapter 2, stem cells are typically harvested from your own abdominal fat, which is lipoaspirated in a simple, office-based surgical procedure. The fat is then processed to yield the stem cell injectate in a process that takes a couple of hours.)

Once prepared, the PRP, with or without stem cells, is injected at the precise location of injury or degeneration and stimulates the body to regenerate the damaged structure. It should be noted that only the patient's own tissues (blood and fat), referred to as *autologous* tissues, are extracted, and therefore no foreign or unnatural tissues/products are ever injected.

An experienced physician may use imaging technology such as an ultrasound to ensure a precise injection into the damaged or deteriorated area. When done properly, these regenerative orthopedic injections are very safe and can yield impressive results with many orthopedic and musculoskeletal conditions.

PRE-INJECTION PREPARATIONS

The American Academy of Orthopaedic Surgeons recommend the stoppage of any medications prior to the procedure:

- Avoid the use of corticosteroid medication for two to three weeks before the procedure.

- Stop taking NSAIDs (nonsteroidal anti-inflammatory medications, such as ibuprofen or aspirin, or anti-arthritis medications such as Celebrex, one week before the procedure. This could include any anticoagulant medications.[1]

FOLLOW-UP CARE

There may be some inflammation and swelling after a PRP treatment is done, but if so, it will be very minimal. Generally, resting and avoiding putting excess pressure on the joint for a couple of days is a good idea. Based on the severity of your condition, a temporary sling for your arm or a crutch for your leg may be suggested post-procedure. This is a precautionary measure for minimizing any undue pressure and stress on the affected joint.

Avoid taking anti-inflammatory medications. The genetic materials in your PRP have the anti-inflammatory properties your body needs, and these natural properties can be disrupted with medications—so let nature have its way. The physician may or may not prescribe something for pain. (I personally have not needed anything for pain, but I have taken arnica and turmeric at different times.) Usually there is minimal swelling at the injection site, which can be cared for by alternating hot and cold compresses for ten to twenty minutes for a couple of days.

The overall experience is very simple, very easily tolerable, and has almost zero aftereffects. Because of the cofactors in the PRP, most if not all of the inflammation you were experiencing is very well dissipated.

Avoid taking anti-inflammatory medications. The genetic materials in your PRP have the anti-inflammatory properties your body needs, and these natural properties can be disrupted with medications—so let nature have its way.

Without a question or doubt in my mind, PRP therapy is something everyone should take advantage of, particularly if you or a loved one is suffering with chronic joint pain or other painful musculoskeletal conditions.

PRP FOR MY NECK PAIN

As I share with you another personal testimonial of my experience with pain and various pain relief treatments, I'm starting to feel like the poster boy for "Who Has the Most Pain." But as I alluded to before, I have lived a very physically active life; consequently, after taking all those hits in football and pushing my body joints beyond human limits in competitive powerlifting, I happen to live with the aftereffects these days.

It was 2009, and I had extremely irritated a preexisting condition in my neck. I was experiencing severe pain that ran down my left shoulder, through my arm, and into my hand and the back of my fingers. It was that searing nerve pain that was almost impossible to bear. The condition immediately caused the loss of 90 percent of the strength in my left arm, particularly in the triceps muscle in my upper arm, including major atrophy (muscle deterioration) of that muscle. I had bulging discs in my cervical spine (neck) and though the pain was felt in the other parts of my body, the pain generator was in my cervical spine at the C–7, C–8, and C–9 joints.

The pain was so intense that I made an appointment to see a neurosurgeon to get an opinion. His office referred me to his radiology department that handled all MRIs and X-rays. After reviewing the MRIs and X-rays, the radiologist said normally they would recommend an epidural injection to reduce the inflammation, but in my case the disc was compressed so tightly and the nerve canal so narrow that an injection would be too risky, and that I needed immediate neck surgery!

The pain caused me to feel nauseated most of the time, and the thought of surgery made me feel even more distressed. So before I opted for surgery, I decided to try a PRP treatment.

I made an appointment to return to the Center for Regenerative Medicine in Miami. My doctor reviewed my MRIs and said he didn't think I needed surgery and was confident that a PRP treatment was all I needed. He performed the outpatient procedure on me and stated that I should come back the following week for a second treatment, which I did. My greatest concern, besides getting some relief from this pain, was a prolonged pinched nerve condition causing permanent damage to the nerve cells.

After I had the second PRP treatment, my doctor said it would take two weeks for the nerve tissue/cells to begin to repair and for the pain to dissipate. Over the next couple of months I did some treatments to my neck every day to enhance blood flow—using my Thera Cane, red light heat, and moist heat pads plus arnica montana, turmeric, and devil's claw (in spite of the terrible name it gets from the tiny hooks that cover its fruit, it is wonderful for pain relief).

It was during those two weeks that I was scheduled to see the neurosurgeon. To my amazement, the pain was subsiding somewhat, but I needed that second opinion. After the doctor reviewed my MRIs, he said I didn't need surgery but he could order an epidural injection. I passed on the injection and went home healed.

And sure enough, by the end of the second week all the pain was gone from my extremities and I started regaining strength and size back to my left arm. Again, I was so impressed with this therapy that I made a conscious decision to always have stem cell and/or PRP treatment(s) before opting for any surgical procedures.

WORD OF CAUTION

One of the major concerns you should have if you are dealing with bulging discs, pinched nerves, or any condition that involves the impingement of a nerve, is permanent nerve damage. Our nerves transport electrical energy to our organs, muscles, and other parts of our bodies to keep them alive and functioning normally. When a nerve is impinged or compressed, the energy force or electrical life is choked out and the organ or muscle tissue will start to prematurely die or lose its normal functionality. This shrinkage of the organ or muscle is referred to as *atrophy*. With PRP therapy (with or without stem cells) the ligaments and tendons surrounding and supporting the spinal joints (vertebrae) are strengthened, which in turn will release the impinged nerve from the bulging disc and preserve the nerve from further damage.

In my travels and appointments, while sitting in the waiting rooms in stem cell clinics, I have personally spoken with men and women of all ages with all types of injuries—even older folks with arthritis or bulging discs in their necks or backs—who have shared with me how their condition improved either during or after receiving stem cell and/ or PRP injection treatments.

When a nerve is impinged or compressed, the energy force or electrical life is choked out and the organ or muscle tissue will start to prematurely die or lose its normal functionality.

As I mentioned before, there is a tendency for most people to gravitate to conventional medical procedures and medicine without considering or being aware of alternatives to mainstream medicine. Alternatives such as PRP and stem cell therapies and treatments are considered disruptive because they are cutting-edge and out of the conventional thinking box. They provide results more quickly, are less invasive, and prevent unnecessary surgeries—and here is the kicker—all by using your own genetic, God-given materials.

So if you are suffering daily with chronic pain and have not found the solution to your problem or are not satisfied with the way your doctor is handling your condition, the information in this book should be very encouraging—there *is* something that can fix your problem. Again, try *everything* else first before opting for surgery.

FREQUENTLY ASKED QUESTIONS

What is PRP, or platelet-rich plasma?

PRP treatment is a medical procedure that was established nearly forty years ago. In the following years, delighted with this new, minimally invasive procedure, doctors tried to apply it to a wide range of conditions in sports medicine, orthopedic surgery, and dental and cosmetic surgery. Platelet-rich plasma is, as the name indicates, plasma that is more abundant in platelets, approximately five to ten times richer than normal circulating plasma.

What is plasma?

Our blood is made up of liquid and solid components. These two parts are *liquid*, which is the plasma, and *solid*, which is made up of red blood cells (erythrocytes, which carry oxygen), white blood cells (leukocytes, which are a part of our immune system), and platelets (thrombocytes, which participate in blood coagulation or clotting).

Why platelets, out of all the cells in our bodies?

The reality is, platelets are not true cells like red or white blood cells. They are just tiny partial cells that originate in the bone marrow and circulate throughout our bodies to prevent us from bleeding out when we get injured. It turns out that in addition to helping blood to clot, platelets carry growth factors—proteins essential for wound healing.

How is platelet-rich plasma prepared for the patient?

It is really a simple procedure. There is an initial blood draw by the phlebotomist. Then the blood is spun in a centrifuge, the spinning effect separates the platelets from other blood components, and a harvesting of the platelets takes place. Once the platelets are collected and mixed with the remaining blood, you have a PRP serum that can be injected into the damaged or inflamed tissue.

How does PRP work?

What we know for now is that growth factors abundant in PRP can potentially accelerate the healing process. The main problem is that this effect varies, so research is under way to try to determine the exact mechanism of PRP and the conditions that can influence this mechanism.

What does PRP cost?

PRP can range in cost from $500 to $1,500. This is not a standard, across-the-board fee or rate, but a range of what I've seen as typical for individual physicians and/or clinics.

Which medical conditions can be treated with PRP?

There are a variety of medical conditions that can be treated with PRP, but with very different levels of effectiveness. The most common conditions are acute ligament and muscle injuries, nerve injuries, cardiac muscle injuries, chronic tendon injuries, osteoarthritis (degeneration of articular cartilage that causes severe joint pain), bone fractures, and even androgenic alopecia (baldness).

There are many new procedures of biological therapy in medicine nowadays, and PRP is one of them. Although promising, there is not sufficient clinical evidence that PRP is effective for a wide range of medical conditions. Most published studies show that PRP is safe to use, but more research needs to be done to determine the overall benefits as well as the potential harm of this therapy. If you are considering a PRP treatment, the safest thing to do is to consult your doctor first. He or she will be able to give you proper advice based on current medical guidelines so you can make the right decision about your health.

STUDIES PROVE THE EFFECTIVENESS OF PRP

Research is now moving beyond trying to prove or disprove the efficacy of platelet-rich plasma therapy as an effective treatment for knee osteoarthritis. PRP *does* work, and this has been made clear by evidence from independent medical researchers.

An example of results from PRP are two new studies from Chinese researchers and one from Thailand that have now been added to the mounting evidence. According to the Get Prolo website, "These studies show PRP injections to be more effective in the treatment of knee osteoarthritis, in terms of pain relief and self-reported function improvement at three, six, and twelve months follow-up, compared with other injections, including saline placebo, hyaluronic acid [HA], ozone, and corticosteroids."[2]

Further current evidence indicates that "compared with hyaluronic acid and saline, intra-articular PRP injection may have more benefit in pain relief and functional improvement in patients with symptomatic knee osteoarthritis at one year postinjection."[3]

The website continues, "Doctors in Thailand published in slightly earlier research that PRP injection improved patient symptoms and function when compared to hyaluronic acid and placebo suggesting that PRP injection is more effective... at reducing symptoms and improving function and quality of life."[4]

Convinced that PRP helps, research is now concerning itself more with trying to explain how to utilize PRP and how it goes about healing knee injuries and knee instability. This knowledge will allow doctors to move forward with treatment recommendations and guidelines.

According to GetProlo.com, "Doctors at the University of California say PRP injections cause positive, beneficial, and healing cellular changes in the joint environment. These changes help move the knee from degenerative knee disease to a healing and regenerating knee joint. Healing includes regeneration of articular cartilage, increasing the volume of natural knee lubricants, and waking up the stem cells present in the knee to assist in the transformation to healing environment."[5]

Researchers wrote: "PRP modulates the repair and regeneration of damaged articular cartilage in the joints and delays the degeneration of cartilage by stimulation of mesenchymal stem cell migration, proliferation, and differentiation into articular chondrocytes (the cells of cartilage)."[6] What this last sentence means is that stem cells in the knees, responsible for repair on many levels, *migrate* (because PRP calls them to the site of the injury), *proliferate* (make more of themselves), and *differentiate* (change themselves into cartilage).

In addition, PRP reduces pain by decreasing inflammation of the synovial membrane, where pain receptors are localized. The synovial membrane is a protective layer of connective tissue that is also responsible for creating synovial fluid that lubricates the joints.

MORE PRP STUDIES

As amazing as the above research is, it is merely one in a progression of studies. Previously, in 2015, the same University of California Davis researchers speculated that PRP provided the lubrication needed to protect the cartilage. The researchers summarized that "intra-articular injections of PRP have the potential to relieve the symptoms of osteoarthritis in the knee and that there is an influence on superficial zone protein (SZP), which is a boundary lubricant in articular cartilage and plays an important role in reducing friction and wear and therefore is critical in cartilage regeneration."[7]

You are fortunate to be living in this day and age where you have these new therapies available to you, because they can offer you a better chance for healing and returning to a better quality of life.

In other words, PRP is acting like hyaluronic acid, except it is healing and regenerating the knee, which hyaluronic acid is not designed to do. HA intra-articular injections are widely accepted for the treatment of pain associated with knee osteoarthritis. The goal of HA viscosupplementation is to reduce pain and improve viscoelasticity of synovial fluid. PRP has also been employed to treat osteoarthritis by possibly inducing cartilage regeneration. The combination of HA visco-supplementation with PRP regenerative properties could supply many advantages for tissue repair.

I hope by now you can see the amazing alternatives and possible options that are available, whether it is stem cell therapy or PRP therapy. Regenerative medicine and these disruptive therapies are changing the old way of "doing business as usual" to new ways with cutting-edge technologies and treatments. I've included the transcript of a one-on-one interview with Helmut Makosch at the end of this chapter because I believe it will both inform and inspire you as you consider stem cell and/or PRP therapy. Over the years I have had stem cell/PRP treatments from both Helmut Makosch in North Florida (Jacksonville and St. Augustine) and the Center for Regenerative Medicine in South Florida (Miami), which is where I received my first stem cell and PRP treatment.

If you are facing a surgical procedure or have a degenerative health condition that has not responded very well and you are still dealing with nagging pain and discomfort through conventional medicine, then take advantage of stem cell and PRP therapies *now*. You are fortunate to be living in this day and age where you have these new therapies available to you, because they can offer you a better chance for healing and returning to a better quality of life.

But with all the good our genetic materials provide for us, there is a concern or awareness I want you to understand. As miraculous and efficacious our natural God-given repair crews—adult stem cells—are, over time our stem cells and cellular health can be challenged. Since we are made up of trillions and trillions of cells and totally rely on their functions to keep us healthy and functioning normally, what can we do when our stem cells need help?

Section 2 will address a couple of hidden questions that beg some answers. For example, what happens when our own adult stem cells begin to lose their ability to repair our cells or their functionality slows down? Is there anything you and I can do to correct the problem without costly treatments, visits to the doctor's office, and a litany of medications?

Since this is a natural degenerative problem and occurs via negative influences like the aging process, illness, disease, trauma, and environmental toxins, everyone is a victim and no one escapes the dilemma—*until now*! So, after you read the following one-on-one interview I conducted with Helmut Makosch, head to section 2 and learn how adult stem cell activators can solve this problem we all face.

My One-on-One With Helmut Makosch

Over the years I have had the opportunity to meet a very impressive person who, in my estimation, is not only brilliant and extremely well-versed as a stem cell scientist but also a caring individual. Since our initial introduction, Helmut Makosch and I have become friends and business associates.

Due to the many TV and radio shows I do, I get people requesting stem cell therapy all the time. I refer them to a stem cell physician I know depending on where in the United States they live. What I typically do is contact the individual and have an initial consultation with them. If they are still interested in stem cell or PRP treatments, then I have Helmut contact them. With his expertise and wisdom, he will spend as much time as needed to explain in detail what he can and cannot do for them regarding their specific condition. From there, the potential patient is free to choose to have treatment or not.

I asked Helmut if he would be willing to sit down and have a one-on-one interview with me to discuss various questions about stem cell therapy, and he said he would! Here is a transcript of that interview.

Dr. Joe: What is your medical training and/or background?

Helmut: Some of my schooling was done in Germany, where I received my bachelor's degree in chemistry, physics, and mathematics and later my MSC in organic chemistry. I became a member of the American Academy of Antiaging Medicine in 2003 and continued my studies in advanced endocrinology, biology, and stem cell technologies. Then

I studied cutting-edge advancements in cell culturing and applications. In 2011 I opened a complete stem cell clinic in Tegucigalpa, Honduras, where we performed the first rebuilding of a heart on a patient given three weeks to live.

Little of what we do can be learned at universities. It is truly pioneer work with patients hands-on that has made SC [stem cell] technologies advance so fast.

Dr. Joe: Do you have a stem cell facility here in the United States?

Helmut: I have two locations...St. Augustine, Florida, and Jacksonville, Florida.

Dr. Joe: What influenced you to pursue regenerative medicine? And for how many years?

Helmut: The greatest influence on me was the success with patients and seeing their tears of joy recovering from hopeless conditions. For ten years I have a history of performing more than one thousand stem cell therapies.

Dr. Joe: Explain the difference between stem cell therapy/treatments and PRP therapy.

Helmut: A platelet-rich plasma (PRP) therapy utilizes a concentrate of growth factors derived from the patient's blood, which when injected into localized areas such as a shoulder, spine, or knee, generally speeds up the healing process significantly.

In stem cell therapy, we use the PRP from the patient to activate his or her stem cells, which have been extracted from the fat tissue utilizing a mini liposuction. The number of cells harvested with our newer technology is typically between five hundred million to two billion cells.

Dr. Joe: What is the typical success rate of SC and PRP therapy with your patients?

Helmut: PRP therapies are often repeated to lead to success while stem cell therapy is mostly a one-time application in orthopedics.

Dr. Joe: Do you specialize in any certain area or areas? Please describe.

Helmut: I specialize in musculoskeletal and degenerative illnesses, arthritis, and sports injuries. Also with diseases such as Alzheimer's, Parkinson's, diabetes type 2, COPD, erectile dysfunction, arthritis, brain trauma, and many more. The most common in orthopedics is shoulders, knees, hips, spine, and neck regeneration.

Dr. Joe: How has SC therapy evolved since you first started?

Helmut: Significantly! We have developed techniques that will yield much greater amounts of stem cells than in the past. We have demonstrated that utilizing 3D printer technology we have regenerated human ears and noses, and that is just the beginning.

Dr. Joe: Where do you see the future of stem cell therapy going?

Helmut: Organs will be cloned and immortal cells will be engineered that may promise a much longer lifespan, perhaps a total reversing of aging and elimination of the aging diseases.

Dr. Joe: What can a patient expect if they come to you for SC treatment?

Helmut: Our success rate based on orthopedic applications is about 85 percent. Many patients are pain-free the next day; however, the actual regeneration process will take two to three months.

Dr. Joe: Is stem cell therapy for everyone?

Helmut: No, it is not for everyone. People with extreme damage to their joints accumulated over years untreated may have reached a point where stem cells are not the best choice. Age, however, is not an issue; our oldest patient was one hundred years old when receiving stem cell therapy.

Dr. Joe: While some treatment centers are administering SC therapy to cancer patients, other people are concerned about the proliferation of cancer cells/tumors if they had SC therapy. Is there a concern or connection with SC therapy and cancer? What are the pros and cons?

Helmut: There is no evidence that stem cells may aid tumors or cancers; however, we do not treat people with these conditions.

Dr. Joe: Is SC treatment successful for antiaging? If so, explain. What areas of treatment?

Helmut: Stem cells given as an IV have, in my opinion, a regenerative effect as reported by many patients. They typically notice improvement to their skin and memory. Since stem cells built our body, they have the potential to repair tissues in most areas of our body and provide more energy.

Dr. Joe: What should an individual look for when pursuing a stem cell clinic/facility?

Helmut: For a consumer, it is important to find a stem cell clinic that has a good success rate and a real stem cell laboratory with a knowledgeable scientist as well as doctors trained in liposuction and injection techniques. Many of the "Kit Systems" [the tools by which the physician provides stem cell therapy] utilized today will not provide enough cells to have enough therapeutic value. It's like sending five thousand troops into battle when thirty thousand were needed.

Dr. Joe: Would you mind sharing a few testimonials of your patients who you treated over the years?

Helmut: I'd be glad to.
  Patient #1—Let's call him Marcus, an old friend of mine. Thirty years ago he had a dirt bike accident. He hit a rock and was catapulted about fifty feet, landing head first in the mud. He barely survived with heavy brain trauma, a triple fracture in his neck including his atlas, broken clavicle, and both shoulders dislocated, as well as lower back injuries. After weeks in the hospital, he was released. His pain was constant and over the years turned into arthritis.
  Marcus ultimately called me, told me that his pain was intolerable, he could not lift his arms to wash his hair, his sciatica was causing also a lot of pain. He stated that he was going from doctor to doctor and several chiropractors with no relief while living on pain medication. Then he

asked me, "Do you think stem cells could help me?"

As a scientist, I must be careful not to promise anything to anyone, because I have very little control over what stem cells will do. I just know that they are powerful and have the potential to repair all kinds of tissues. I told Marcus based on what I have witnessed stem cells do, I would do therapy ASAP. Marcus came all the way from Canada and was treated in a five-hour procedure. The harvest of total stem cells was over 1.2 billion cells with over 96 percent viability. All his ailing regions were injected. He also received an IV to target lung inflammation [for which he had been] treated for twelve years. His arms' range of motion improved overnight by 26 and 76 degrees respectively. The second day after SC therapy he was pain-free and his lungs had completely cleared as well.

Marcus told me he wished his doctors would have known about SC technology. He went back to work and had a new life as he stated. Since I cultured his cells, he came back four years later to have a booster IV with his own cells and states that he feels great.

Patient #2—Let's call him Walter. Walter had previous open bypass surgery of the heart and two stents placed. Years after this intervention Walter's heart caused trouble again; this time his right ventricle of the heart was in necrosis (the heart muscle was dying). His wife (an angel) called me, crying, "I don't want to lose my husband. The cardiologist gave him about three weeks to live.... Isn't there anything you can think of to save my husband?"

I replied, "Yes! I can think of a possibility, but it has never been done before."

She said, "Let's do it..."

We took a biopsy from Walter's thigh muscle to run a culture.... We needed his own muscle cells to stop the necrosis since his SC would take about twenty-eight days to differentiate. We were up against time.

I took Walter to my clinic in Honduras to harvest his SC and started an additional culture with his cells for future therapies. At the medical center, I had a team of two cardiologists, a special heart anesthesiologist, and seven assistants. Walter's SC and muscle cells where injected via special catheter directly into various regions of his heart. This was five years ago. Walter is alive and doing well.

Patient #3—Let's call him Mr. Smith. Mr. Smith had

stage 4 Crohn's disease. Vanderbilt University and Mayo Clinic gave him an estimated three months to live. His pain was extreme and he would get up at three in the morning to prepare his body for work at 9:00 a.m. Mr. Smith took $11,000 worth of medications per month.

When I started his SC treatment and parallel cultured his cells, he quit all medications cold turkey. Mr. Smith was given an IV of his stromal vascular fraction (SVF) of over 1.5 billion cells. Within days he noticed a rapid decline in pain and inflammation. I further treated Mr. Smith in a protocol containing six more treatments from his culture. Even though Mr. Smith eats all the wrong foods for his previous condition, he has no symptoms.

After four years Mr. Smith went back to Vanderbilt University, where he was tested utilizing a capsule camera that travels through his intestines. His doctors where baffled as they compared old images to this new one and stated, "We can't find any Crohn's. What did you do?" Mr. Smith is now almost six years free of this disease without medication (a big loss to Pharma).

SECTION II

Adult Stem Cell Activation

W HEN OUR STEM cells are functioning properly and normally, all is well. They can go about their business of repairing tissue and cells and keep our body functioning normally. But there are questions that beg to be asked:

- What do we do or what can be done should their ability to repair become disrupted or impaired?

- If our adult stem cells cannot signal or communicate with one another normally, then what domino effect will occur?

- Will there be a detrimental impact to our health?

- What if one cannot afford to pay for stem cell treatments? Is there a more affordable option that is still effective enough to radically change one's health?

In this section we will address all these concerns. We will take a close look at what you and I can do to revitalize our own adult stem cells (our natural cell repair team) when they have become impaired or lost their ability to signal or communicate to one another. You will learn just how simple, natural, and efficacious the results are as you revitalize your own stem cells by simply "activating" them. In fact, adult stem cell activation is, in my estimation, another disruptive technology for repairing, restoring, and rejuvenating tissue and cells in our bodies.

As we move on through this section, I'll explain what adult stem cell activation is and how it works. I'll also explain the technology behind the targeted adult stem cell activators I've been using, plus their many benefits and possible applications for health-related problems such as sports injuries, accidents, chronic diseases, depression, insomnia, memory loss, attention disorders, autism, degenerative conditions, obesity, diabetes, chronic fatigue, arthritis, organ disorders, and many, many more.

You will also read some of the many testimonials that my office staff receive from people who have started taking adult stem cell activators. We learn from their feedback that they are no longer in constant pain, are experiencing fewer and fewer degenerative illness issues, and not having to make numerous doctor visits and blood work appointments like they once did. Their testimonials are very encouraging and exciting.

As you learn from the materials I am sharing with you, I hope that through this book you will be better informed and educated about adult stem cell activation so you can make wiser decisions concerning your personal health issues—those nagging, painful, uncomfortable health issues that never seem to disappear. Ultimately, I want you to begin experiencing that greater quality of life that has been missing for such a long time.

CHAPTER 4

ACTIVATING DAMAGED ADULT STEM CELLS

I DON'T KNOW ABOUT you, but I find these disruptive technologies and adult stem cell therapies extremely fascinating. Learning all about what adult stem cells are, what they do for our bodies, and the therapies and treatments that are available today has taken regenerative medicine, restoration, and healing of the body to the next level. Should you ever require adult stem cell therapy, the reality of what I am saying will make a true believer out of you—no doubt!

From a non-scientist perspective, my goal has been to provide for you a better understanding of the importance and function of our adult stem cells. We now know they repair our bodies' tissues and cells, they can differentiate or become another cell type, and they can restore and rejuvenate damaged tissue so we can avoid certain surgical procedures and degenerative diseases.

STEM CELLS CAN HEAL AND REGENERATE:

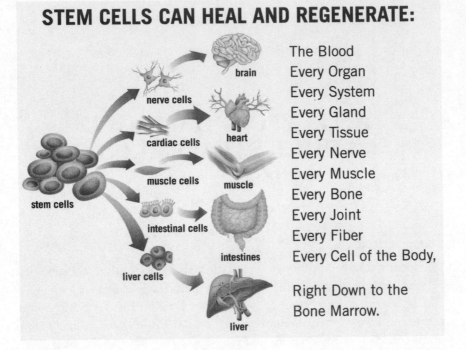

The Blood
Every Organ
Every System
Every Gland
Every Tissue
Every Nerve
Every Muscle
Every Bone
Every Joint
Every Fiber
Every Cell of the Body,

Right Down to the
Bone Marrow.

In section 1 we learned that this built-in cell repair and renewal crew was given to us at birth and is a part of our genetic makeup. Should any of our organs, bodily systems, or bone tissues become damaged or destroyed, our stem cells step up and hone in on the specific damaged body parts and begin their repair work. Adult stem cells actively work to help replenish our bodies with their own innate or natural process. When they are performing their duties, our bodies should be functioning at their optimum.

But what happens when adult stem cells stop or slow down their function due to natural causes or conditions out of our control? I've already covered the disruptive treatments available through stem cell therapy and PRP therapy, but what if an individual cannot afford these disruptive treatments? Is there an alternative?

The answer is yes, and to better prepare you for any misfortune with your health, allow me to assist you by educating you on the topic of adult stem cell activation so you can have a firm foundational understanding of these natural miracle workers.

In the process, I'll explain how I came to learn about a very effective way for everyone to reap the benefits of stem cell activation: by taking adult stem cell activators. I'll explain the science behind adult stem cell activators so you will have more confidence in them and be better equipped to make an educated decision. Should the moment arise when you or a loved one requires attention to your health and physical condition, being up on adult stem cell activators and what they can do to correct your condition will be priceless.

But before we start, let me now share with you some of my own personal health challenges and victories I have experienced by taking adult stem cell activators.

ACTIVATING MY ADULT STEM CELLS

Just before I open my personal data to you, please allow me to set the record straight regarding getting positive results. Whether a technology, therapy, nutritional supplement, or any modality or protocol has scientific and/or medical support to prove its efficacy or not, *one cannot argue with the reality of results!*

As you have probably realized by now, the stem cell treatment approaches I'm discussing in this book, while used by a growing number of physicians, are not widely used yet, and therefore, some in the medical community have not yet accepted them. This is also true in the case of the stem cell activators, which many would categorize as alternative or natural medicine. I've reviewed clinical research conducted on the activators that is not available to the public as of yet. Until it is, I can wholeheartedly recommend the activators based on my clinical understanding as a naturopathic doctor and on the experiences of myself and others. Of course, the medical community will downplay any results that one may have experienced that have happened outside of their conventional box and medical journals. Whether the results are the matter of healing a dysfunctional organ like the pancreas or kidney or correcting a degenerative illness, they view them as merely being anecdotal. Well, this is where I must disagree with the conventional mentality.

When a patient tells me they are off dialysis since taking adult stem cell activators or they are no longer experiencing joint pain or neuropathic pain and/or numbness in their feet since taking stem cell activators, I don't think anyone has the right to say their experience is merely anecdotal. Oh, and by the way, this is a perfect example of the difference between the mind-set of conventional medicine and that of those embracing what disruptive technologies and therapies are doing for mankind.

OK, let me get back on track and share my own personal testimonial with you. I have had wonderful results with adult stem cell activators. In my case, being intuitive with my body and how it responds, I can easily tell if something I take works or if it does not work at all. For me, the litmus test was my ailing and painful shoulder ligaments that had been intensifying in pain for some time. You may relate to what I am referring to with regards to painful shoulders if you or someone you know have been told by an orthopedic physician that the crippling pain you're experiencing is coming from a partially or full-blown rotator cuff tear, which is a tear in the tendons/ligaments, also called connective tissue.

As I mentioned, I have always made daily exercise a vital part of my life. But the shoulder pain I was experiencing was so horrific that it drastically limited the amount of weight I could lift and eventually got to the point where I had to discontinue exercising for a while. I was also experiencing limited range of motion in my shoulders. But the story doesn't end there.

Inflammation and pain go hand in hand, and my shoulder ligaments were interfering greatly with everything I did. They hurt during the day while driving my car or sitting at my desk, even restricting my ability to raise my arms high enough to brush my teeth. When it came to bedtime, forget about it! A full night's sleep was impossible. As a matter of fact, the simple motion of pulling a bedsheet or bedcover over me was incredibly painful.

Even with all the pain, I was not about to settle for a surgeon to perform an arthroscopic procedure on my shoulder with hopes of repairing some damaged ligament tissue—at least not before testing every therapy, treatment, and technology first!

Before You Choose Surgery...

Here are a couple of considerations for anyone opting for surgery. There is never a guarantee that the problematic areas will be fixed, but there is the possibility of the procedure being botched. At best there are the residual effects of scar tissue buildup to keep in mind, as well as the amount of time to recover, and any possible added inconvenience and discomfort if you have to wear something like an arm sling. After all that, you may end up over time still living with a certain level of pain. Surgery was not my first choice of defense, nor should it be yours.

Please don't misunderstand me. If you've had surgery in the past, my goal is not to condemn you or make you feel bad about it. I'm sure you made the best decision you could based on the information you had at the time. It's likely that you fully understand the downsides of surgery that I'm talking about if you have experienced any of them since electing to have that surgery. My point is, by reading this book, you are arming yourself with new information and giving yourself new options for anything you currently face. It's a new day, and regardless of what has happened in the past, my goal is to open your eyes to the new options you now have instead of surgery.

OK, so you say, "What should I expect from my body at sixty-nine years old, right?" Wrong. Listen, I may be sneaking up on seventy, but to me, age is just a reminder to keep living my life to its fullest potential with purpose and relevancy. I have a mind-set that accepts nothing less than doing all I can do to ensure a life of optimum quality. Unless you have settled for allowing your age or current health condition to determine your quality of life, *now* would be the perfect time to start doing something about it!

Of course, I was given the typical conventional remedies and protocols for rotator cuff injuries and pain. I combined minimum conventional medicine and maximum alternative medicine approaches to see if I could correct the problem. I tried a mild dosage of medication for the inflammation and pain but vowed that I would not use it for too long. I bumped up my intake of natural anti-inflammatory supplements such as turmeric and arnica (homeopathic remedy). I applied ice and heat therapy and red light therapy, rested the area, got some physical therapy, and even made some lifestyle adjustments.

Symptom stompers (anti-inflammatory medications or pain medications) can help as a quick fix for the short term, but they should never be considered for long-term use because they can never heal a problematic area in your body.

That pretty much sums up the best that you and I can ever do to hopefully repair and restore any problematic area back to normal function. After implementing all these remedies, if we happen to hit the jackpot in the process, we can rid our bodies of all symptoms and our injured body parts are prepped for healing. For a while, my shoulders did start to heal—until I used them. Then the pain returned and I went back to square one.

After repeating the same protocols several times over and over, I found that the symptoms would not go away for long, so I kicked around the idea of having an arthroscopic procedure done, but then decided not to. As I said earlier, even with all the pain, I knew there were other therapies and treatments that were available outside of that conventional box—disruptive therapies!

Enough with treating symptoms! Sure, symptom stompers (anti-inflammatory medications or pain medications) can help as a quick fix for the short term, but they should never be considered for long-term use because they can never heal a problematic area in your body. The best line of defense when it comes to healing our bodies, alleviating pain, and getting back to normal function is to eradicate the *root cause*. If you have been treating symptoms by taking meds for months or even years, you had best make some serious changes before the root cause of your condition becomes irreparable.

I knew I could have another stem cell treatment, but I wanted to test this new adult stem cell activation technology I had been researching. When I found there were adult stem cell activators I could take at home without having to travel to a clinic or doctor's office, I was even more convinced they were a great option. Plus, unlike stem cell treatments, the activators were very affordable by anybody's standards.

There are twenty-six different adult stem cell activators available, each one targeted to a different organ, system, or tissue of the body, such as the kidneys, pancreas, adrenal glands, nervous system, and others. I selected the activators targeted for connective tissue since the ligaments in my shoulders were painful and inflamed. By the way—using the activators targeted for the connective tissue meant other ligaments and soft tissue in my body would benefit also!

> *If you have been treating symptoms by taking meds for months or even years, you had best make some serious changes before the root cause of your condition becomes irreparable.*

As I was taking the activators every morning throughout the first month, I was looking for some level of relief if possible. Let's keep in mind I still exercised every day (though limited), which in and of itself would normally slow down any improvement. Prior to taking the activators, I was not able to lift my arms over shoulder height without feeling a high level of pain and was forced to take a break from exercising.

After making that adjustment from my workouts within those first thirty days, I found myself able to perform exercises that involved my shoulders that I had stopped doing, and I noticed very little pain. My day-to-day activities became less and less painful. I could go to bed and not be woken every few hours by the pain in my shoulders. I could tell things were improving nicely.

I continued taking the activators for a second month. I noticed that I could increase my exercise workout load and that nagging, lingering pain that had previously been present after my workouts was gone. I knew I'd found the remedy to my painful shoulders. Not only had my exercise program progressed, but my life in general was back to being normal and enjoyable and pain-free again.

I learned that a pattern of taking the activators every day for three to six months and then taking a break from them to reevaluate my shoulders worked best for me. I also knew I would continue exercising, which would put an additional strain on the ligaments. That's why I prefer taking the activators every day, which is the accurate regimen for the physical workload on my shoulders and physical lifestyle.

The logic behind this protocol of taking the activators was based on my physically active lifestyle and my chronic shoulder condition. Just those two factors alone made me realize it would behoove me to continue activating the adult stem cells in my ligaments.

The results have been that I can exercise regularly again and enjoy living my life in general without having to contend with nagging pain and discomfort—all things I couldn't do prior to taking the adult stem cell activators!

Because I experienced such amazing results, I'm passionate about sharing this information with you. That's why I've written this book. But before we delve into this fascinating phenomenon of activating our damaged adult stem cells, let me share with you what—or should I say *who*—inspired me to further embrace this concept that I already found to be both efficacious and promising, both on a personal and professional level.

I'm sure you have experienced at some point in your life that one special person who seemingly played a major role in certain events or critical periods. Whether that individual was instrumental in helping you make the transition to a new chapter in your life, or encouraged you to make that business choice, or was there just to bounce your ideas off, each of us could identify that one person. It's that one person who was the catalyst for positively affecting our lives at the most pivotal time. In my case, that person was my mother!

MOMENTS WITH MOM

One day in early 2015, I was having a talk with my ninety-year-old mother about her visits to the two doctors who were treating her failing kidneys and dysfunctional pancreas (for diabetes). The physician who was treating her kidneys with medications due to her diabetic condition had just explained to her that her kidneys were now down to only 25 percent function. He then went on to tell her that if they continued to drop in function, his prognosis for her was to be placed on dialysis. He highly suggested she begin preparing herself and her family members for the likelihood of starting weekly dialysis treatments in the near weeks and months to come.

To say my mother was terrified by the prospect of having to be hooked up to a dialysis machine for three days a week would be an understatement. I could tell by the look of fear on her face and hopelessness in her voice that the reality of her current health status looked more like a death sentence rather than offering any future glimpse of hope!

Well, I was not about to allow my mother and lifetime champion and cheerleader go down without a fight. I told her that there was a disruptive technology that I believed strongly in that might correct the problems she was having with both her pancreas and kidneys. I told her I could not promise this concept would work, but at that point, all that was being done for her was only treating her symptoms. She had nothing to lose but so much to gain, so I introduced her to the concept of what adult stem cell activation was all about.

I began by explaining to her the role adult stem cells play in her body and their association with her overall health, and how they were responsible for repairing damaged cells in the body. I explained that my strategy was to go to the root cause of her failing kidneys instead of treating the symptoms only. We all know that treating symptoms will never correct a failing health condition, organ dysfunction, or failing bodily system.

I told her that her kidney adult stem cells were not functioning normally because they were somewhat compromised and damaged and needed to be repaired. Consequently, the kidney cells themselves were apparently damaged. This cellular damage was most likely the root cause of her failing/damaged kidneys while being induced by an underlying condition—diabetes. I mentioned that as we age, our adult stem cells can take longer to do their job even in the best of conditions, when disease or illness is not present.

But also, on the other hand, one's adult stem cells can lose their ability (cellular signaling) to repair various cells throughout the body due to illness, disease, trauma, environmental toxins, and even the aging process. Because of the health conditions she was experiencing—diabetes and failing kidneys—plus factoring in her age, the adult stem cells themselves needed to be repaired and rejuvenated.

After this brief explanation, I went on to tell her that our goal was to activate her adult stem cells for her kidneys and pancreas. We would do it naturally by having her take adult stem cell activators just like I had done for my shoulder. I explained to her that these adult stem cell activators were targeted and designed for specific adult stem cells found in the various organs, bodily systems, and tissue throughout the body. (I'll provide a full list of all the activators and explain their applications in chapter 6.)

I started her regimen with two different types of activators. One was targeted for her kidneys, and the other was targeted for her pancreas. I explained how to take them daily, and like a good trouper, over the next several months she followed my directions and took them every day religiously.

It was approximately three months later when she had a follow-up appointment with both physicians and wanted to tell me about the results. As she shared the good news with me, I could sense a heightened level of excitement in her voice that was so opposite of how discouraged and helpless she felt when she learned the bad news from her doctor only three months earlier.

She started sharing with me what the physician who was treating her diabetes told her. Prior to taking the activators for her pancreas, her A1C numbers were dangerously elevated to 11 and needed to come down.*

Lantus was the insulin medication her physician had her inject daily. Though it helped support and regulate her sugar levels, it only served as a bandage at best and would never be able to cure or restore her pancreatic function. Consequently, her condition worsened over the years, and considering her age, any improvement of her diabetic condition was most unlikely.

But to her doctor's amazement and surprise, my mother's A1C had dropped a couple of points, from 11 to 9, which never happened with medication. Because of the improvement, he wanted to reduce her current insulin unit injections by 50 percent. This improvement was quite amazing, especially since it occurred in such a short period of time. Her physician said he didn't know what was going on but told her to keep up the good work.

Right about this time in her story, I was jumping up and down. First, because this patient was my mother; and second, because my mother was responding quickly to what the activators are designed to do! Of course, other variables like managing her diet and staying physically active and exercising had to be factored in—but *wow*, was I thrilled!

Then my mother told me the wonderful news about her kidneys. Her physician had been elated with the results and was happy to report that her kidneys had *not* gotten worse. In fact, not only did they seem to be stabilizing, but they appeared to have *improved*.

Keep in mind, not only was her age a factor but also the fact that she was diabetic. These were the two major contributors that worked against her physiology. With the mind-set in conventional medicine, continued degeneration of the kidneys would be the norm at her age, even with the use of medications. There would be no expectations or

---

* One's A1C test measures how well the body is handling the glucose (blood sugar) in the blood by assessing the amount of what is called *glycated hemoglobin*. An A1C level below 5.7 percent is considered normal. Prediabetic signals are when the A1C is between approximately 5.7 and 6.4 percent. Type 2 diabetes is diagnosed when the A1C is over 6.5 percent.

even a remote chance for kidney improvement for someone like my mother. To me, that can be a death sentence for anyone who is not informed. But for my mother, that changed because of the adult stem cell activators.

Her physician went on to say that he didn't feel it was necessary for her to receive dialysis treatment at that point but said they'd see how things went over the next few months. Instead of having to prepare herself and her family for the dreadful nightmare of having to go on a dialysis machine, she could finally relax because she felt there was hope.

I can't tell you how thrilled and relieved I was as I listened to her level of excitement and relief from the fear of going on dialysis. To know my mother was out of the woods, so to speak, made all my research, application, and implementing of adult stem cell activators worth the time and effort.

Shortly before I completed writing this book in the early fall of 2017, my mother passed away as she approached age ninety-three. If you didn't read my dedication to her at the beginning of this book, written shortly after her death, I encourage you to look at it now. Although Mom suffered from heart failure, diabetes, and kidney disease, I am thrilled to report that for the last two and a half years of her life, while she faithfully took the adult stem cell activators, her kidneys did not drop in function and remained stable, allowing her to evade dialysis that entire time.

By going to the root cause and activating and rejuvenating her kidney adult stem cells, they in turn began doing their job of repairing her kidney cells. Her kidneys stopped declining in function and began functioning more normally, and Mom dodged the dreaded bullet of dialysis treatment.

Even though she passed away two and a half years later from complications of multiple conditions, as I ponder how baffled her renal physician was by the improvement of her kidneys, I can't deny that her results from taking these adult stem cell activators were not only an answer to our prayers—they were nothing short of a miracle!

BEING REALISTIC

You need to realize that none of us are the same, and therefore, neither will the results we experience be the same. There are many factors to consider when it comes to the healing and rejuvenation process of problematic areas in our bodies. After all the factors are considered—age, overall health, severity of the condition, type of condition, and length of problematic areas—my initial recommendation to anyone considering taking adult stem cell activators is to allow for a minimum of three months before reevaluating your condition. The reasoning is simple.

When taking the adult stem cell activators, we graduate the dosage up to the maximum amount within a few days (instead of months like medications). For most people, three months of continual daily intake of activators being transported by the blood to the targeted areas provides significant serum levels for repairing and restoring the damaged adult stem cells.

Let me make this perfectly clear: I am not saying that it takes a minimum of three months before one experiences any improvements. As a matter of fact, my office staff is flooded with reports from our patients and customers who tell them that they notice improvements within a few days and weeks. But from my professional perspective, to ensure the repairing and rejuvenating of the individual's adult stem cells I prefer a three-month minimum start for developing a good base to build on. After that, the individual can reassess their condition and decide if they should continue more adult stem cell activation, reduce the amount, or discontinue all use because the problematic area has been corrected.

ACTIVATORS FOR PERIPHERAL NERVE PAIN

I recall a cruise Lori and I had been on. We happened to be in the fitness center talking with someone when I noticed a woman moving closer and closer to our conversation. When we finished our conversation, this woman introduced herself and said she couldn't help but hear what we were talking about—of course, what stem cell activators are and how they work.

She went on to tell us she had Morton's neuroma, a condition that made walking very painful for her feet. Morton's neuroma is a thickening of tissue around the nerve between the bases of the toes. Foot pain and numbness over the ball of the foot are common symptoms. The condition makes normal walking very difficult. She was forced to wear flat shoes instead of high heels because it made the pain more tolerable, but nevertheless walking was still a painful experience. She went on to say that her doctor prescribed medications, which she claimed did not help at all. She had experienced two failed surgeries and now was living with constant pain.

After returning home, I called her on the phone and shared more information about adult stem cell activators with her. Based on what she shared with me, I explained that it was apparent that she had damaged nerve tissue that needed to be repaired so it could heal. I went on and told her about a specific adult stem cell activator that was targeted for neuropathy or peripheral nerve pain. I felt that specific activator would best meet her needs. She ordered two bottles, approximately a two-month supply.

I did a follow-up call two months later to see how she was doing. She told me that within those first two months, 90 percent of her pain was gone. The numbness was almost gone as well. She told me she could start wearing her high heel shoes again, which she couldn't do previously. (FYI—high heel shoes contribute to Morton's neuroma, so I don't recommend this.) How could I argue with her results?

REPAIRING MY NERVE ADULT STEM CELLS

My personal experience with the activators did not stop there. To be totally candid and transparent, I must admit that this old battleship of mine (my body) has had some very tough sailing over the years. Today I am paying for its journey in terms of lingering joint pain and nerve pain from the damage I caused to my body during my competitive body-building days. This nerve pain is sometimes referred to as neuropathy.

Neuropathy or neuropathic pain is a complex, chronic pain state usually accompanied by tissue injury. With neuropathic pain, the nerve fibers themselves may be damaged, dysfunctional, or injured. These damaged nerve fibers send incorrect signals to other parts of the body. This was the case with the woman I just spoke about.

Because of my previous back surgeries, today I still experience numbness in my left thigh within minutes of standing. I also experience nerve pain in certain areas of my feet. There are times when a couple of my toes on each foot go numb and times when they are painful. This condition is not rare as many people suffer with nerve pain or what is referred to as neuropathy.

This condition may be the result of someone being injured in a severe auto accident, taking a hard fall, or from sports injuries to the back or neck that traumatized the athlete's spine. Then there are those who may be genetically predisposed to spinal deformities and experience nerve pain problems in their extremities. This damage to the spine is directly correlated to peripheral nerve damage.

Since I was convinced of the efficacy of the activators, I started taking the activator targeted for peripheral nerve damage, which is directed at the adult stem cells in the nerves. In just three or four weeks I noticed at least a 50 to 60 percent decrease in pain and discomfort in my feet. I take this activator daily because my greatest concern is permanent nerve damage or the inability of nerve conduction to go to my extremities. When permanent nerve damage occurs, the area of the body connected to the nerve experiences a loss of energy, which could translate into *organ atrophy* (premature death of the organ), loss of motion, or movement to another area where the nerve sends its energy.

An example is what is referred to as a "floppy foot." The causes of floppy foot are a spinal injury, stenosis, narrowing of the nerve canal in the spinal column, or a severely pinched nerve from degenerative disc disease. The root cause is in the spine, where the nerves are being impinged and therefore incapable of properly, if at all, sending the electrical energy to the foot. The longer the nerve impingement remains, the greater the chances of permanent nerve damage. Consequently, if the impinged nerves are those that go to the feet, then the person starts experiencing the loss of *dorsiflexion*. Dorsiflexion is when you tap your toes up and down on the floor when listening to music, or when you lift your foot as you take steps while walking. It is obvious that the sooner one can repair and rejuvenate the nerves, the greater the chances of avoiding permanent nerve damage—something that should be avoided at all costs.

With modern advancements in regenerative medicine like stem cell therapy, some of these degenerative conditions that have been treated conventionally can now be repaired and restored to normal function. Similar results can happen when taking adult stem cell activators.

There is an interesting phenomenon about these activators—and in this case, the peripheral nerve activator. Because it helps repair and rejuvenate the adult stem cells in the nerves in my lower back/lumbar spine, the repaired nerve cells can then function normally and send electrical energy signals to my legs and feet. When that happens, the nerve damage is repaired, the neuropathic pain and numbness in my legs and feet dissipates, and I can enjoy my life again.

Now should I have an area of my physiology that needs attention, I can immediately use the appropriate activator(s) to repair the adult stem cells at the root cause, which in turn helps restore the problematic area back to normal function.

If you are suffering with neuropathy, nerve pain, or peripheral nerve pain from damaged nerve cells/tissues, then I highly recommend that you consider this adult stem cell activator. As I mentioned, there are many modalities in which we can try to manage our painful conditions, but if all we are doing is masking the symptoms, then you and I have zero hope of experiencing lasting improvement.

For over two and a half years my mother experienced positive results from taking the adult stem cell activators. At the time of her passing at age ninety-three, she was doing just fine and had never had to go on dialysis as was once prognosticated. Since I have continued having positive results over the past three years, plus the many reports and testimonials of patients of mine who share their positive results and improvements, I felt very compelled to share the activators with everyone I encounter.

I am very confident, excited, and passionate about adult stem cell activators and their efficacy because I know what it is to be in chronic (and/or acute) pain without an option other than medications and/or surgeries. In the next chapter I'll explain the science behind these activators and what makes them amazingly safe and effective.

CHAPTER 5

THE SCIENCE BEHIND ADULT STEM CELL ACTIVATORS

Throughout this book I purposely have been candid and transparent by revealing some of the health concerns that I contend with on a day-to-day basis. I hope my personal stories serve as a means of encouragement to you and assure you that whatever you are struggling with regarding your health, you are not alone by any means. At times you might feel like you are facing your pain, fear of the unknown, or uncertainty about what to do all by yourself, but this book should help you realize that there are others facing the same obstacles—and, more importantly, there is hope for a brighter tomorrow where you can leave the pain and fear in the past!

Though at times my personal journey can sound a bit painful and challenging, I make it a point to strive in overcoming any health issues I have or might have in the future by taking advantage of the disruptive therapies and technologies that are available. This adult stem cell activation approach is both preventative and reactive in nature. It allows me to minimize or eliminate any painful or inflammatory conditions or possible degenerative illnesses so I can ultimately reach and maintain the greatest quality of life possible. Because of my unwavering willingness to never quit using the disruptive therapies and technologies I have mentioned in this book, my stories have also included the victories I am experiencing.

In addition to my personal health stories, I felt it necessary to share with you the personal health conditions of my mother regarding her kidney dysfunction and diabetes, and her miraculous results since she started taking the adult stem cell activators. The reason is, again, to make you aware of these disruptive therapies and embrace their advanced restorative properties. Should the need arise for something more advanced than the treatment options you have had in the past, you will be prepared to maximize your results.

Unlike in the past, there are new answers for the physiological and degenerative health problems that cause many to suffer. Therefore, please keep an open mind and willing spirit!

Now let's consider the science behind the adult stem cell activators with which I've been involved.

THE SCIENCE

Our bodies are comprised of hormones, blood, neurotransmitters, muscles, and organs—all combinations of *amino acids*, the building blocks of life. These amino acids combine into chains to form peptides and proteins, out of which countless numbers of the cells that form all body tissues and organs are made. All problems within our bodies start when communication between these cells begins to break down due to harmful elements in our environment, an unhealthy lifestyle, or diseases.

Unlike embryonic stem cells, the adult stem cells are present in all tissues of the human body from the moment of birth.

All cells interact with each other through a system of control signals, which are passed from one cell to another via the bloodstream, the body's main information carrier. Once cells receive this information, they "know" what to do. All biological processes, whether genetic instructions, cellular division, metabolism, or even cellular death, are strictly controlled by these regulatory signals. This process is known as *regulatory transduction*. If these signals are not "heard" by the cells, or if they pass through distorted (imagine static on a telephone), the processes governing the cells run out of control, which leads to all sorts of health hazards, such as organ dysfunction or tumors.

Fortunately, our bodies already have a built-in source for cellular regeneration: adult stem cells. These cells are best viewed as a renewable cellular reserve. They do not have the cellular structure of a tissue or organ but can be activated and converted to such specialized structures. The primary role of adult stem cells in a living organism is to maintain and repair the tissues and organs in which they are located. Unlike embryonic stem cells, the adult stem cells are present in all tissues of the human body from the moment of birth.

Definition, Please!

Nanotechnology is the science and engineering concerned with the design, synthesis, and characterization of materials and devices that have a functional organization in at least one dimension on the nanometer (one-billionth of a meter) scale. In other words, it deals with matter so small, it's on an atomic or molecular scale. "One-billionth of a meter" might be hard to imagine. If you took a human hair and divided its thickness into eight hundred equal parts, one of those parts would be close to the size of the matter being researched and manipulated in nanotechnology.

NANOTECHNOLOGY

In over fifteen years of research, scientists have discovered that certain *regulatory peptides* are naturally secreted by the cells of various body tissues in response to cellular damage to activate adult stem cell conversion. However, this process occurs very slowly, even under the best of circumstances. If the cellular trauma is severe enough, this very mechanism of cell regeneration gets damaged and doesn't work fast enough—or in the worst case, it doesn't work at all!

ProtoMedix scientists, utilizing *nanotechnology*, have created regulatory peptide-based nanoparticles for use as active ingredients in the adult stem cell activators.[1] A unique quality of these nanoparticles is that they are active in ultra-low doses (ULD): 1 gram (0.035 oz.) of the active ingredient is sufficient for sixty million full strength doses. Once introduced into the body, nanoparticles reestablish optimal communication between the existing cells and activate adult stem cells of targeted organs to start rapid conversion and replacement of damaged cells. Because these particles are thousands of times smaller than individual cells, active in ultra-low doses, and naturally present in the human body, they do not cause any side effects or allergies.

As I mentioned, these adult stem cell activators contain regulatory protein-based nanoparticles that are created utilizing nanotechnology and are unavailable as part of any other product on the world market today. One of the powerful qualities of these nanoparticles is their *bioactivity*. Bioactivity basically means influencing a living organism, tissue, or cell. Other examples of bioactive substance are antibiotics, enzymes, and vitamins.

These nanoparticles are structured with a regulatory protein core surrounded by lipids and carbohydrates. They provide stability and protection from the destructive influence of various enzymes, including digestive enzymes of the gastrointestinal tract. Without this unique structure, the digestive enzymes would destroy the efficacy of the activators. Once introduced into the body, these active nanoparticles easily pass through the intestinal walls, enter the bloodstream, and are carried to the tissues or organs for which they were formulated.

Because these particles are thousands of times smaller than individual cells, active in ultra-low doses, and naturally present in the human body, they do not cause any side effects or allergies.

Upon reaching a targeted organ or tissue—say, for example, the kidneys—these nanoparticles mimic the body's natural processes, reestablishing optimal communication between the existing cells. Once this occurs, the adult stem cells start rapid conversion and replacement of the damaged cells. The damaged cells are then naturally absorbed by the body, leaving the tissue or organ healthy once again.

The extraordinary potential for healing and repairing tissue and cellular damage that this disruptive natural therapy could do for others became obvious to me through my own personal experiences and results. The potential for restoration and recovery from injury, illness, and many other conditions is now much more possible, more convenient, and more cost effective than many of the common modalities that have been available thus far in my professional years.

ACTIVATING MY OWN ADULT STEM CELLS

As mentioned earlier, I have experienced stem cell and PRP therapy many times. I've had treatments on my lower back, hips, and neck. In fact, the most recent treatment was on my lower back in June 2017. I had been moving a lot of furniture and household items at my mother and father's house for nearly three months. After all that bending, stooping, and lifting, my lower back had all it could take. The muscle spasms were severe, and the pain in the sacroiliac (SI) joint was preventing me from getting a full night's sleep. Even lying down in certain positions was painful.

I had applied several of the common protocols to my back (ice and heat packs, body massages, some gentle stretching) but to no avail. In desperation, I decided to make an appointment with a local chiropractic clinic for an evaluation and possible treatments. After the initial evaluation, X-rays, and consultation, I was scheduled for two weeks of treatments and adjustments to remedy the problem. As it turned out, the root cause of my problem was beyond the reach of the treatments I was receiving. Within those two weeks, nothing improved. I was still in constant pain and knew I needed to take a trip to see my stem cell physician.

I needed more than a tune-up; I needed an overhaul. So I took another trip to Miami to see my doctor at the Center for Regenerative Medicine. The trip from Orlando to Miami is approximately a four-hour drive, and it was difficult to sit for so many hours. I could not get comfortable because of the pain, so consequently I had to make several pit stops along the way.

It was worth the discomfort because the stem cell procedure was simple but methodical. First the phlebotomist drew my blood, which was then placed in a centrifuge to separate the plasma, growth factors, and stem cells. Then my doctor performed a mini liposuction and extracted the stem cells and the adipose tissue (fat cells) from my abdomen and prepared the combination for stem cell treatment. The PRP/stem cell combination using autologous stem cells (my own stem cells) was a perfect treatment and seemingly exactly what the doctor ordered—no pun intended. Then after some therapy, I was sent on my merry way.

Now for the acid test—the long drive back to Orlando. Would I notice an immediate improvement or not? Well, as I suspected (prayed for), the trip was comfortable and I needed no pit stops. After arriving home, within the first twenty-four hours, 90 percent of the pain and discomfort was gone. Within the first week, my lower back felt much more relaxed, the level of pain had subsided, and I was back to being my normal self. The outcome of the stem cell treatment couldn't have come at a better time. As it was, Lori and I were only a couple of days away from boarding a cross-country flight from Orlando to Seattle for a fourteen-day cruise in Alaska. Any of my apprehensions about lower back pain ruining our long overdue vacation had been resolved.

Here's a tip: the goal of healthy living is not to see how much pain and discomfort you or I can endure over time, but rather to live with as little pain as possible!

Yet you may be thinking to yourself, if stem cell therapy and PRP therapy are all that great, then why have it done repeatedly? Without sounding redundant, not everyone is the same nor responds the same way to stem cell treatments. There are several factors to consider, such as the severity of injury or joint damage, the level of pain, and the person's age and physical condition. Various degenerative conditions could require more treatments than other conditions that are acute in nature. Sometimes there are multiple problems and/or areas that need treatment.

In my case, my spine is unstable due to many past sports injuries and trauma to my spine. If you want to add the back surgeries I have had into the mix, it is obvious to see how easy it is for me to experience severe muscle spasms, sciatic nerve pain, and neuropathy—thus my need for an overhaul from time to time.

But there's one thing I would like to convey to you: it is better to take advantage of stem cell therapy sooner rather than later. As you well know, many of us tend to suffer long with our conditions and put off any form of medical treatment until we can't stand the pain any longer.

Here's a tip: the goal of healthy living is not to see how much pain and discomfort you or I can endure over time, but to live with as little pain as possible!

I have made daily exercise a part of my healthy lifestyle choices (I will discuss the aspects of a healthy lifestyle later in section 3), but back in the day, it was a different story. Back then I was eyeballs deep in competitive powerlifting and bodybuilding and grueling workouts during which I beat my body beyond reason. Imagine pushing and pushing this body to go beyond what it was designed to do while in constant pain just to win that trophy or title.

If the only residual effects from all that insanity were just the sore muscles and stiffness in my joints, then that would have been easily relieved with proper stretching, reduction in intensity of exercise, and spending more time to relax and allow the muscles and joint tissue to recover. But unfortunately my joints, spine, tendons, and ligaments have the lingering long-term negative effects from competitive sports and training that I pay for today.

As efficacious as the results that I have had with PRP therapy and stem cell therapy are, some conditions remain a nagging hurdle to overcome and sometimes require day-to-day maintenance or at least special attention.

Researching new modalities, treatments, advanced technologies, and nutrition-based protocols has always been my motivation so I can best serve my patients and my family members as well as myself. Having to deal with a nagging, painful hurdle of my own really pushed me to research more and more, which ultimately brought me to the most advanced natural treatment or protocol I could find—adult stem cell activators.

I needed something natural that could improve my overall joint health and mobility. I needed something to lower or eliminate pain so I could not only participate in regular exercise but simply enjoy life without carrying an ice pack everywhere I went. I needed some technology or natural modality that could support healing, eradicate the root cause of my pain, and ultimately even provide a cure.

Now hold on a minute! Did I just say *cure*?

I would ask you to forgive me for using "the C word," but being the eternal optimist, I cannot. I cannot disregard the possibility that somewhere out there in a laboratory are ongoing experiments, trials, and tests with various remedies, modalities, and technologies whose end game is finding a cure. Excuse me if I am enthusiastic about healing, repairing, and rejuvenating my (your) body back to normal and healthy functionality, even at the expense of stumbling on a cure along the way!

BENEFITS AND POSSIBLE APPLICATIONS

Establishing healthy cells is where the rubber meets the road. The foundation to your overall health and wellness starts at the cellular level. It has been long known that no matter the original cause, whether lifestyle excesses, environmental toxicity, injury, or disease, all body tissue breakdowns begin at the cellular level.

The ability to control cellular regeneration within the damaged tissues is an increasingly important focus for many researchers worldwide. The scientists who pioneered this field over forty years ago and are behind the scientific data for the adult stem cell activators published the first article in 1976.

It's what takes place at the cellular level that has the greatest influence on our physiology. It is necessary for proper digestion and assimilation of the nutrients from our food as well as the elimination process.

Optimum cellular signaling (communication from one cell to another) is imperative for repairing and restoring damaged cells and tissues to proper cellular function. The health of our cells is directly related to many benefits, such as reducing and even eliminating chronic pain and degenerative illnesses.

Benefits and Possible Applications of Adult Stem Cell Activators

Let's look at some of the benefits and possible applications that adult stem cell activators have to offer.

Benefits:

- Speed recovery from injury and surgery
- Minimize scar tissue formation
- Enhance cardiovascular performance
- Activate immune defense system
- Modulate an overactive immune response
- Enhance metabolism and detoxification
- Normalize blood sugar metabolism
- Enhance brain function and mental state
- Improve neurological conditions

- Aid in weight management and fat metabolism
- Support endocrine hormone balance
- Improve digestion and absorption
- Increase energy, endurance, and resilience
- Improve oxygen supply to organs
- Promote recovery of overexerted organs and tissues
- Sharpen concentration and memory

Possible Applications:

- Sports injuries
- Chronic diseases
- Depression and insomnia
- Memory loss and attention disorders
- Autism
- Degenerative conditions
- Obesity
- Diabetes
- Chronic fatigue
- Arthritis
- Thyroid disorders
- And many more...

Without a doubt, this technology is very encouraging and exciting and brings plenty of hope to those who are struggling with various illness and poor health conditions. Now let's take a deeper look into these adult stem cell activators to get a better understanding of what it means to be "targeted" for specific organs and systems in the body.

CHAPTER 6

TARGETED ADULT
STEM CELL ACTIVATORS

I FIND IT VERY fascinating that the adult stem cell activators I've been involved with are targeted. They will travel through the bloodstream directly to the organ or tissue at the root of the patient's problems, bypassing the destruction of the intestinal enzymatic actions, where they would normally lose their strength for healing and repairing. The macronutrient coating and the nanotechnology allows them to avoid the destruction so they can repair and restore the damaged adult stem cells at full strength. As we know, once the adult stem cells have been rejuvenated and repaired, they can perform their duties and repair the damaged cells in the body.

So with that understanding, let's look at a list of twenty-six adult stem cell activators that have recently been developed for targeted applications. See if you can identify any areas of your health that need help and which activators are targeted accordingly.

TWENTY-SIX TARGETED
ACTIVATORS AND RELATED AREAS*

1. Adrenal support (SC-ADR)
Regulates intercellular communication and supports cellular and tissue regeneration in the adrenal glands of the body; able to render regulatory influence on the adrenal gland hormones. Possible applications

---

* For product availability, go to www.bodyredesigning.com or call 1-800-259-2639.

for adrenal dysfunction/insufficiency, fatigue, exhaustion, salt balance, blood pressure, and metabolism imbalance.

2. Bladder support (SC-BLDR)

Regulates intercellular communication and supports cellular and tissue regeneration in the bladder. Possible applications for bladder tone, incontinence, urinary urges, and bladder issues.

3. Blood sugar support (SC-Blood Sugar)

Regulates intercellular communication and supports normal blood sugar levels. Possible applications for blood sugar imbalances, fatigue, weight gain, nerve and vision issues, and metabolic syndrome.

4. Blood support (SC-BLD)

Regulates intercellular communication; supports cellular and tissue regeneration in the cardiovascular system and supports blood homeostasis, oxygenation, and immune function; has ability to render regulatory influence on development and functioning of T and B cells. Possible applications for infections, degenerative and pathological conditions, endothelium, anemia, hemorrhoids, arterial wall damage, varicose veins, and more.

5. Breast tissue support (SC-BRST)

Regulates intercellular communication and supports cellular and tissue regeneration of the breast. Possible applications for degenerative and pathological breast conditions, hormone and glandular conditions such as ovarian cysts and degeneration, menstrual irregularity, inflammation, and more.

6. Cellular support (SC-ONC)

Regulates intercellular communication and promotes apoptosis. Possible applications for apoptosis and uncontrolled malignant cellular activity.

7. Central nervous system/brain support (SC-CNSE)

Regulates intercellular communication and supports cellular and tissue regeneration in the central nervous system (brain); supports cognitive and neurological function and stimulates efficiency of central nervous system. Possible applications for strokes, dementia, depression, anxiety, psychiatric issues, overstrain of nervous system, weariness of eyes, and more.

8. Central nervous system/nerve support (SC-CNSN)

Regulates intercellular communication; supports cellular and tissue regeneration in the central nervous system. Possible applications for neurological degeneration, amyotrophic lateral sclerosis (ALS, also called Lou Gehrig's disease), multiple sclerosis, complex regional pain syndrome (CRPS, also called reflex sympathetic dystrophy or RSD), neuropathy, nerve damage, degenerative and pathological conditions, and more.

9. Connective tissue support (SC-CNT)

Regulates intercellular communication and supports cellular and tissue regeneration in the connective tissues of the body; helps protect cells from toxic action and has great potential in gerontology. Possible applications for toxicity, viruses, sex organs and gerontology, sports injuries, hernia, sagging skin, prolapsed uterus, scarring, stretch marks, ligaments and tendons, and more.

10. Endocrine system support (SC-ENDO)

Regulates intercellular communication and supports cellular and tissue regeneration in the endocrine system; optimizes hormone balance for both men and women. Possible applications for hot flashes, menopause and andropause symptoms, premenstrual syndrome (PMS), adrenal fatigue, pituitary insufficiency, infertility, sperm motility, cysts, erectile dysfunction, libido, and more.

11. Female hormone balance (SC-FEM)

Regulates intercellular communication and supports cellular and tissue regeneration of the female endocrine system. Possible applications for disorders of the female reproductive system and endocrine system such as menstrual disorders, fertility issues, ovarian insufficiency, depression, and more.

12. Gallbladder support (SC-GB)

Regulates intercellular communication and supports cellular and tissue regeneration of the gallbladder; optimizes gallbladder function. Possible applications for degenerative and pathological gallbladder conditions such as sludge, gallstones, fat metabolism, bile insufficiency, and more.

13. Heart support (SC-HRT)

Regulates intercellular communication and supports cellular and tissue regeneration in the heart and cardiovascular system. Possible applications for coronary and valvular heart conditions, arrhythmias, history of myocardial infarction, heart failure, cardiomyopathy, and more.

14. Hypothalamus support (SC-HYP)

Regulates intercellular communication and supports cellular and tissue regeneration of the hypothalamus; it can render regulatory influence on the endocrine system. Possible applications for deep emotional issues, hormone balance, autonomic nervous system issues, body temperature issues, adrenal and pituitary issues, salt and water balance, sleep issues, eating disorders, iron imbalances, growth issues, and weight and appetite imbalances.

15. Optimal weight support (SC-OPTIWEIGHT)

Supports homeostasis in the hypothalamus; balances the hunger response; restores transmission of information on the status of fatty reserves; helps normalize motor activity of bowels and improves digestion; stimulates binding and removal of toxins from the body; assists in purification of the blood and lymph; helps normalize microorganisms of the bowel; strengthens digestive, immune, nervous, and cardiovascular systems; encourages detoxification and prevents premature aging. Possible applications for reducing excessive body mass index, and normalization of fat and carbohydrate metabolism.

OptiWeight

I thought it necessary to touch on the topic of weight loss. Most people who have a weight loss goal eventually find it difficult to achieve, at least from a lasting perspective. They gravitate from diet to diet (see chapter 8) in their eagerness to find the one that works. But most people soon discover it is not as simple as diet. There are more areas that need to be considered for successful weight loss, and of course, it starts at the cellular level.

Obesity has become one of the biggest health problems of the twenty-first century. More and more young people become obese these days. Obesity contributes to the development and progression of serious health problems such as heart disease and diabetes.

We know that excessive food consumption plays a significant role in the development and progression of obesity. However, this only becomes possible with the disturbance of functional connections in the cell(s) when changes appear in the passage of the information signal, which corresponds to the maintenance of a constant body mass. When the activators, which are herbal/plant-based regulatory peptides, are combined with nanotechnology, they directly reactivate cellular signaling, which in turn stimulates hormones, the brain, and the hypothalamus.

The OptiWeight activator is aimed at reducing excessive body mass index, normalization of fat and carbohydrate metabolism, improvement in the function of organs that regulate digestion, detoxification, and prevention of premature aging. Right now you're probably reading this and saying, "That's great, Dr. Joe, but exactly how does it work?" Allow me to explain.

The high efficiency of this activator is confirmed by the results of clinical experiments and gives an unusually powerful effect.

OptiWeight actively stimulates *leptin* synthesis (leptin is a hormone that regulates a feeling of fullness). This initiates the transfer of information about energy reserves to the brain and causes the activation of the hypothalamic center. This in turn regulates appetite and contributes to the reduction in the activity of the lipoprotein *kinase* in the body's adipose tissue, which leads to reduction of fat and eventually participates in the transmission of information into the hypothalamus about the state of fat reserves. Leptin regulates the level of the neuropeptide Y hormone, which increases appetite and contributes to a rise in the mass of visceral fat.

The OptiWeight activator normalizes the activity of the endocrine system, stimulates the pancreas function, possesses diuretic action, helps the liver and kidneys, helps with heart and nephritic edemas, contributes to an improvement in microcirculation, and contributes to the hydrolysis of the cellular reserves of fat and removal of toxins from the intercellular space. It also increases bile secretion, decreases the content of bilirubin, accelerates metabolism, actively stimulates digestion, decreases appetite, and dulls a feeling of hunger. The high efficiency of this activator is confirmed by the results of clinical experiments that I have reviewed but are not yet available to the public.

Notation—Weight loss is stubborn for some people, and many times it is due to underlying problems in the endocrine system. As a proactive measure, I will recommend the addition of the ENDO activator to accompany OptiWeight. ENDO, which works for both men and women, will help cellular integrity and cellular repair in the endocrine system.

16. Immune system support (SC-IMN)

Regulates intercellular communication and homeostasis in the immune system and supports the body's natural defenses; effective immune modulating factor for autoimmune diseases. Possible applications for autoimmune conditions, lupus, Hashimoto's disease (thyroid), ITP platelet disorder, and more.

17. Kidney support (SC-KDN)

Regulates intercellular communication and supports cellular and tissue regeneration in the kidneys; enhances fluid regulation and detoxification. Possible applications for toxicosis, degenerative and pathological kidney conditions, nephrosis (kidney disease) with protein in the urine, low blood protein levels, high cholesterol levels, swelling, chronic anemia, chronic fatigue, kidney failure and insufficiency, high blood pressure, recurrent kidney infections, dialysis support, edema, and more.

18. Intestinal tract and digestive support (SC-LGI)

Regulates intercellular communication and supports cellular and tissue regeneration of the digestive tract and mucosa. Possible applications for degenerative metabolic and pathological disorders; inflammation such as colitis, leaky gut; functional intestinal disorders such as irritable bowel syndrome (IBS), constipation; intestinal enzyme deficiencies, and more.

19. Lung support (SC-LNG)

Regulates intercellular communication and supports cellular and tissue regeneration of the lungs and bronchial tubes. Possible applications for chronic pulmonary infections, pneumonia, bronchitis, emphysema, fibrosis, other degenerative metabolic and pathological conditions.

20. Liver support (SC-LVR)

Regulates intercellular communication and supports cellular and tissue regeneration in the hepatic system. Supports body's natural detoxification process. Possible applications for hepatitis and other degenerative conditions of the liver, treatment of new abnormal tissue growths, oncological conditions, and more.

21. Pancreas and digestion support (SC-PANC)

Regulates intercellular communication and supports cellular and tissue regeneration in the pancreas. Supports body's natural ability to regulate blood sugar. Possible applications for pancreatitis, diabetes support, pancreatic insufficiency, degenerative and pathological conditions, and more.

22. Pituitary gland support (SC-PIT)

Regulates intercellular communication and supports cellular and tissue regeneration of the pituitary gland. Possible applications for thyroid issues, endocrine imbalances, muscle imbalances (one muscle is stronger or weaker than its opposing muscle), kidney imbalances, and growth hormone irregularities.

23. Prostate gland support (SC-PROST)

Regulates intercellular communication and supports cellular and tissue regeneration of the prostate gland. Possible applications for prostatitis, prostate hypertrophy, and other pathological and metabolic process disorders.

24. Skeletal/bone support (SC-OST)

Regulates intercellular communication and supports cellular and tissue regeneration of the bones. Possible applications for osteopenia, osteoporosis, rickets, fractures, and other degenerative and pathological bone conditions.

25. Thymus gland support (SC-THYM)

Regulates intercellular communication and supports cellular and tissue regeneration in the thymus gland and immune system. Possible applications for microbial and viral infections, degenerative and pathological conditions, and more.

26. Thyroid gland support (SC-THYR)

Regulates intercellular communication and supports cellular and tissue regeneration of the thyroid gland. Possible applications for degenerative and pathological thyroid conditions, and more.

TAKING YOUR STEM CELL ACTIVATORS

How to take the stem cell activators

Everyone is unique, as is their condition, but there is a base, so to speak, to build upon when it comes to taking the activators. I recommend starting with five to seven drops for the first few days. Then titrate up a few drops daily to the full dose of twenty drops per day. (Remember, we can graduate to the maximum dosage much faster with these activators than you might typically be able to do with medications prescribed by conventional doctors.)

A typical daily dosing is something like this:

- Days 1 through 5, take 5 to 7 drops per day

- Days 6 through 9, take 10 to 15 drops per day

- Day 10 and on, take 20 drops per day

Put the activator drops into two to three ounces of water. If possible, take them on an empty stomach upon first rising in the morning. You can take up to four different types of activators but *do not* mix them together. You must allow fifteen to twenty minutes in between taking them. This also applies to intake of food, beverages, medications, and supplements. The spacing allows for maximum absorption and assimilation.

> *Unlike some medications, it is not necessary to take the activators for the rest of your life. As your body responds to the activation, you may determine whether you prefer to continue usage or discontinue.*

Should your condition be chronic, and if you are over fifty years of age, you can start with a full twenty drops per day. Do not exceed twenty drops per activator at one time. There is no proven advantage in exceeding that amount. (For some very chronic conditions, fifteen drops in the morning and fifteen drops in the evening may be suggested.)

Adult stem cell activators are natural, so there is no harm in taking them for long periods of time. However, unlike some medications, it is not necessary to take the activators for the rest of your life. As your body responds to the activation, you may determine whether you prefer to continue usage or discontinue. It is a matter of what your body is telling you to do or not to do! (As I mentioned in chapter 4, some people have reported feeling a difference within days or weeks; however, I recommend taking the drops for a minimum of three months before reevaluating your condition.)

The activators contain regulatory peptides (amino acids—building blocks for protein) obtained from natural sources using nanotechnology, which reestablishes cellular communication and activates adult stem cells. These preparations are nontoxic and do not cause allergic responses in long-term applications. The activators are intended to support the body's natural processes. They are not intended to diagnose, treat, cure, or prevent any disease.

TESTIMONIALS—ADULT STEM CELL ACTIVATORS

To me, nothing says it better than the testimonial of someone who has personally experienced healing, restoration, and improvement from a painful condition, degenerative illness, disease, or problematic health condition. I encourage you to view these testimonials as *real people* who have obtained *real results*—because that's exactly what they are! Hopefully, their experiences will further encourage and inspire you to try everything as you pursue better health and quality of life.

Shingles

For many years I had been living with a slow burn type pain. Having had shingles, the pain was unbearable at times. I heard about stem cell activators and purchased the CNSN for nerve pain. Almost immediately after taking them, it was like the pain was "unplugged"! I have no pain, especially in my feet. I'm doing great and have no more pain.

—PATRICIA FROM FLORIDA

Kidney donor transplant list

My daughter has kidney failure and was placed on a kidney donors transplant list. We heard about the stem cell activators and decided to try them for her kidneys. After two months of taking the KDN activator, the doctor said she could be taken off the kidney transplant list because of apparent improvement of her kidneys.

—ANONYMOUS FROM FLORIDA

Congestive heart failure

We took my husband by ambulance to the hospital due to severe shortness of breath. He was quickly diagnosed with congestive heart failure and three blocked arteries to his heart, and as they said, he was on death's door. He was admitted and they wanted to do open heart surgery right away, but the doctor was not available. I started using the HRT stem cell activator for the heart immediately along with Total Nutrition plus, Micronized Vitamins and minerals to support the heart and body along with the PTL II laser to support him. He became quite stable after the first twenty-four hours and continued to get stronger. The surgeon wanted to send him home because he was doing so well, but his cardiologist insisted we remain in the hospital for the next ten days awaiting surgery because, as he said, he almost died.

They did an echocardiogram which showed his ejection fraction was only at 30 percent and normal is around 50 to 55. They also did a heart cath which showed the three blockages— one was completely blocked and two were 80 percent blocked.

They said due to lack of blood flow the lower part of the heart appeared to be dead or dormant, but hopefully once the surgery opened the blockages and blood flow was restored then maybe the lower part would operate again, but maybe not at full capacity. Also, they found one valve was leaking and said it would have to be repaired. He also had an aortic aneurism that would have to be repaired with a graft. As you see, it was not good.

So, during those ten days we gave him daily the HRT to activate the adult stem cells of the heart, we also gave him good nutrition and used the PTL II laser on him all daily. After his open-heart surgery, his doctor came out and told me he did amazing and that it was very odd—the valve that showed it was leaking in the test was completely normal. He also did amazing during recovery and had very little pain.

We continued to use the HRT activator daily. We were told that he would always be in congestive heart failure, but when they did his echo six weeks after surgery, they were in shock and could not believe that his heart was functioning at normal level and his ejection fraction was at 50 percent now. He has continued to be their star patient. As a support, we still have him take the HRT several times a week to support his heart. He now leads a very normal life at seventy-one.

—Debbie from Atlanta

COPD

I've had COPD for over twenty years. I took the activators for my lungs and in two months had an examination. My pulmonary doctor told me that my lungs were clear. That was the first time they were clear in twenty years.

—Carl from Canada

Diabetes

Diabetes runs in my family, and so I have diabetes like my mother and sister. I heard about stem cell activators on TV. I was so desperate for answers that I thought I would give them a try. I am pleased to say that my A1C dropped from 8.5 down to 6.5.

—CAROLYN FROM OMAHA

Walking miracle

An 84-year-young woman! I am a walking miracle. I was a nurse for many, many years but struggled with nerve pain, bladder issues, and osteoarthritis. Since I have been taking the activators, I have mental clarity, lack of pain, blood vessels look great, and I feel younger than I was before! I am so delighted with the results.

—RUTH FROM ARIZONA

Pain-free joints

I have been dealing with RA (rheumatoid arthritis) for over ten years. My knees were so sore and my joints were full of arthritis and pain. I started the CNT and [in] only two weeks or so they are doing miracles with my joints. My knee and joint pain is almost all gone and I sleep much better. Thank you.

—MISS WILLIAMS FROM MIAMI

Ulcerative colitis

I was twenty-seven years old and found myself hospitalized for three weeks due to a severe colon condition. I was told I probably needed to have my colon removed. I went home and started on the LGI and the CNT adult stem cell activators. Within a couple months the pain and discomfort disappeared. I did not need surgery and am doing amazingly well.

—SHIRLEY FROM TUCSON

Lyme disease

I had been treated for Lyme disease for a long time and had severe nerve pain and bodily malfunction. Once I started taking the CNSN, I got great relief.

—CARL FROM CHICAGO

Kidney disease

Being on dialysis for months and on a kidney transplant list can make anyone afraid of their future. After taking the stem cell activators for my kidneys, I eventually came off dialysis. Thank you so much for your research.

—KENNY FROM SAN DIEGO

Diabetes

I had met with Dr. Joe and told him about my bouts with diabetes. He told me to start taking these stem cell activators for my pancreas. I had to call him to let him know within the first week I woke up fully refreshed, had lots of energy, and felt better than I had in fifteen years. I ordered my second bottle and can't wait to see my blood sugar test results.

—JOHN FROM NEW YORK

Weight loss

After taking the OptiWeight, I have lost eight pounds in just three weeks. I am so excited about what this seems to be doing to my body. I understand it is repairing many systems, so I'm looking forward to its full effect.

—DONNA FROM NEW YORK

I have found that it has taken me a bit longer than I expected with the OptiWeight, but after a month of consistent use as directed I started losing about three pounds a week. I can't wait to see where I can go with this.

—ELLEN FROM BOSTON

I love this product. When I feel I need to drop a few pounds, I use the OptiWeight. My body responds very quickly, and I can drop those pounds very quickly. I can tell my digestion and elimination is definitely improved, so I am assuming this has contributed to my weight loss.

—CHERYL FROM DALLAS

THE TOP FIVE DEGENERATIVE
ILLNESSES AND CONDITIONS

I wish I had the space to write the personal stories we get in my office every day from callers who are suffering with degenerative illnesses, musculoskeletal pain and inflammation, and other health conditions. It is so heartbreaking to listen to these men and women who are at a loss as to what to do with the neuropathic pain in their legs or feet as nothing they've tried has helped. Or the person with joint pain, knee pain, or back pain so intense that they are unable to do most things they used to do. Or those who are emotionally stressed with fear of not finding something that can help them. Last but not least, those who have lost hope in living because their poor health has literally crippled their quality of life!

But the good news is that while I cannot guarantee results or promise a cure, I can offer hope! My experience in working with my patients taking adult stem cell activators has proved to be nothing less than extraordinary. I get constant reports of people who come in with severe hip pain or joint pain and within a few days, weeks, or months, they are pain-free. Others with neuropathy, lung disorders, or kidney or liver problems find major improvement—the list goes on and on.

I decided that for the next few pages I will target five of the most common conditions for which my patient database seeks help so that you or someone you know can get a better understanding of the options you have to heal quicker, be out of pain sooner, and experience a better quality of life!

1. Pancreas/pancreatitis

The pancreas, a large gland behind the stomach next to the small intestine, functions in two ways:

1. It aids digestion by dumping powerful enzymes into the small intestines.

2. It releases two hormones, glucagon and insulin, into the bloodstream to assist the body in controlling the use of energy from food.

Damage to the pancreas can happen when digestive enzymes are activated, attacking the pancreas gland before they are released into the small intestines. When your pancreas becomes inflamed, it is referred to as pancreatitis. There are two types of pancreatitis—acute and chronic.

- **Acute pancreatitis** is a sudden inflammation of the pancreas for a short period of time. It can range from mild to severe and even life-threatening. Some people can recover from acute pancreatitis with the correct treatment, but when the condition is severe, there is tissue damage. This condition can cause serious harm to other vital organs such as the heart, kidneys, and lungs.

- **Chronic pancreatitis** usually lasts much longer than acute pancreatitis. In most cases, it appears later in life with severe symptoms as a result of alcohol consumption over the years.

Symptoms of severe pancreatitis
- Pain radiating into the back from the upper abdomen
- Nausea and/or vomiting
- Fever
- Tender-to-touch stomach
- Swollen stomach
- Tachycardia—increased heart rate

Causes of severe pancreatitis
- Long-term alcohol consumption
- Gallstones
- Medications, trauma, infections
- Metabolic disorders and surgery

Adult stem cell activator for the pancreas
In most cases of severe and chronic pancreatitis, the underlying damage to the tissue/cells is of great concern and must be addressed. This condition is due to trauma, infection, toxicity, or medications, which in turn can damage the pancreas adult stem cells.

Of course, there are conventional measures—meds to relieve pain, remove blockage to the ducts, and surgeries—that can help the patient.

But I have found that when an individual takes adult stem cell activators, their symptoms begin to dissipate. The pancreas adult stem cells have been repaired and rejuvenated. Once that occurs, these natural repair crews can repair the pancreas cells, and the end result is a pancreas that returns to normal function.

As I mentioned, chronic pancreatitis can affect the heart, kidneys, and lungs as well. People with diabetes, heart issues, and even lung issues can really benefit from taking the targeted adult stem cell activators for each organ or gland (PANC/pancreas, LNG/lung, KDN/kidney, LVR/liver).

Testimonial

> My husband is a diabetic. He had been taking medication for his disease. When I heard about the adult stem cell activator products, I was very curious. So, in June 2017 we ordered one bottle of PANC for his pancreas. He took twelve drops per day until he went through the bottle. His doctor was very pleased with his blood sugar number reduction today (August 2017). He will be ordering more bottles. Thank you.
>
> —JOYCE FROM NORTH CAROLINA

2. Musculoskeletal pain

It's easy to spot the two root words—*musculo*, referring to our muscles, and *skeletal*, referring to our skeletons or bones—indicating that this system is comprised of tendons, ligaments, bones, joints, and muscles. Every movement, the body's stability and support, and even the body form itself is part of the musculoskeletal system. Our joints are supported and stabilized by ligaments, and our bones are connected to muscles by tendons. The musculoskeletal system is made up of this connective tissue or soft tissue.

This connective tissue has no blood or oxygen flowing to it and consequently takes forever to heal and repair. It's easy to see how falls, auto accidents, sports injuries, trauma, and degenerative conditions not only leave one with lingering, nagging, painful inflammation but also limit the ability to move around properly, disrupting one's entire life.

Symptoms of musculoskeletal pain

Musculoskeletal pain is often associated with a specific joint or area of the body, such as the lower back or neck, but some individuals feel pain all over the body, like they overworked themselves shoveling snow after the first snowfall, or they might have an achy feeling in the muscles after being a "weekend warrior." Sometimes one can feel fatigued and tired, especially if the pain is interfering with the ability to get a deep, restful sleep. The most common symptoms are pain, fatigue, and sleep disturbances.

Causes of musculoskeletal pain

Musculoskeletal pain can be caused by accidental falls, trauma, overuse (work and/or sports or exercise), poor posture, sedentary lifestyle, auto accidents, and tight muscles.

Adult stem cell activators for musculoskeletal pain

To relieve inflammation and pain, conventional medicine offers various therapeutic protocols such as ice and heat, massage, physical therapy, anti-inflammatory and pain medication, and eventually surgery. Although these can be effective at times, they do not go to the root cause—cellular damage.

On the contrary, our patients attest to experiencing tremendous results by taking specific or targeted adult stem cell activators. Because the activators are targeted, one can select the specific activator needed (for example, the OST activator for bone/joint issues and CNT for connective tissue such as ligaments and tendons). By doing so, the activation power repairs the adult stem cells in the bones, ligaments, and tendons, and therefore the inflammation is reduced or eliminated and the pain subsides or is eliminated. The damaged cellular tissue is now repaired and the body returns to normal function again.

Testimonial

Five years ago, after returning from a mission trip, my hip and leg were hurting all the time. I limped when I walked, and at eighty-seven, I didn't know what to do. My doctor said I needed a hip replacement operation, but I didn't want one. I tried everything but nothing worked. I saw Dr. Joe on TV and I wanted to try the adult stem cell activators he talked about.

After taking five bottles, the CNT and OST, I do not limp anymore, no more pain, and my leg is much better. I feel fantastic. I have been healed!

—NADIA FROM WEST PALM BEACH

3. Neuropathy/neuropathic pain

The term *neuropathy* refers to any damage, disease, or trauma that happens to nerves. Neuropathy is classified by the area(s) in which an injury or damage has occurred. It can also be classified by disease, as in the case of diabetic neuropathy.

Types of neuropathy

- Peripheral neuropathy is sensory nerve tissue damage that occurs outside of the spinal cord and brain, affecting the nerves of the extremities (legs, feet, toes, arms, hands, and fingers).

- Proximal neuropathy is damaged motor nerve tissue located in areas such as the shoulders, buttocks, hips, and thighs.

- Cranial neuropathy is damage to the nerves that leave the brain. Two common types are optic neuropathy (pertaining to nerve signals to the eyes/vision) and auditory neuropathy (referring to the nerves signaling to one's hearing abilities).

- Autonomic neuropathy refers to damaged nerve tissue of the autonomic (involuntary) nervous system, which includes the heart, blood pressure, blood circulation, digestion, bowel movement, and even sexual arousal.

Symptoms of neuropathy

- Peripheral neuropathy—tingling, numbness, pain that travels to extremities

- Proximal neuropathy—muscle weakness, atrophy (muscle tissue loss), muscle paralysis

- Cranial neuropathy—vision issues, blurred vision, macular disease, cataracts, loss of hearing, ringing in the ears

- Autonomic neuropathy—bowel and bladder problems, possible heat intolerance; sometimes an underlying condition may be involved.

Causes of neuropathy

Causes include diseases, infections, vitamin and mineral deficiencies, autoimmune disorders, alcoholism, heavy metal toxicity, toxins, injuries/trauma, and drugs and medications. As you can see, these are all directly related to what destroys and damages our adult stem cells.

Adult stem cell activators for neuropathy

Unfortunately, most conventional medicine treatments for nerve damage range from medications such as carbamazepine (for epilepsy) to antidepressants to opiates (pain medications). Medications like these are what I call "symptom stompers" that don't address the root cause and create toxicity and major side effects. Some even have addictive properties.

Instead of treating the symptoms, though that may be helpful in the short term but never works long-term, I believe in going to the underlying cause—damaged adult stem cells. When we activate the damaged adult stem cells, they are rejuvenated and repaired and able to repair the damage to the nerve/nerve systems.

When a patient is dealing with cognitive issues such as vision or hearing problems or a brain injury, I recommend the CNSE activator for brain or cranial neuropathy. Those who have nerve pain in their feet, toes, legs, buttocks, shoulders, arms, hands, or fingers, the CNSN activator works best. The results are less or no nerve pain, reduced or eliminated numbness, improved muscle strength and size, and better overall bodily function and mobility.

Testimonial

[I] had lived with pain in my feet and toes for years. My doctor diagnosed me as having Morton's neuroma. He performed two surgeries which did nothing but caused more pain and difficulty in walking, plus medications that didn't work. I spoke with Dr. Joe about his activators for nerve pain and he said to take the CNSN activators. Within two months 90 percent of

my pain and numbness has disappeared. I can walk with zero
pain for the first time in years.

—Mary from Texas

4. Gallbladder pain

The gallbladder, located near the liver, stores a fluid called bile from
the liver. Even though a person can live without a gallbladder, it plays
an important part in proper digestion. I personally have never imag-
ined our Creator giving us an unnecessary part like the gallbladder. Oh
yes, you can live without one, but there are consequences.

When a person becomes acidic or develops acidosis, the body naturally searches for alkaline minerals to balance its own pH. The gallbladder steps up and utilizes the bile salt as one form of alkaline
mineralization to counterpunch the high acid level in the body. But
when the gallbladder has been surgically removed (cholecystectomy),
the body will divert to another place in the body (e.g., the bones) to
leach calcium, another alkaline mineral—and the domino effect begins.
In many cases, when a person restores or balances his or her pH, the
symptoms from the gallbladder dissipate. One important side note—an
acidic environment is the perfect environment for cancer to grow.

Symptoms of gallbladder pain

Symptoms include a painful feeling between shoulder blades and/
or under the right rib and sometimes nausea and even vomiting.
Abdominal discomfort and pain will often intensify after eating a meal,
especially a meal that is heavy in fat.

Causes of gallbladder pain

When cholesterol in the gallbladder forms into stones and passes into
the small intestine or gets caught up in the biliary duct, it causes a lot
of pain. (Liquefied cholesterol becomes hardened like stones because of
its acidity.) Of course, alcohol consumption and diet can contribute to
pain as well.

Adult stem cell activators for gallbladder pain

I prefer going right to the root problem—the cellular damage that
was either causing the condition or caused by the condition. In either
case, I have received wonderful reports from those individuals who

have had severe gallbladder attacks and found relief when taking the activators.

Because the activators are targeted, I suggest the GB activator as the place to start. When the solidified cholesterol turns into stones, the sooner one can pass them, the better. By repairing the adult stem cells, they in turn can repair the gallbladder cells, and ultimately the probability of future attacks is greatly lessened. Keep in mind, lifestyle plays a huge role in this as well. (See section 3.)

Everyone should exercise regularly or even daily, eat accurately for their blood type,* stay hydrated, reduce stress levels, take on a positive attitude, take time to play, and get away from the grind. Healthy lifestyle practices (see section 3) are essential for all types of treatments and therapies whether conventional, regenerative, or alternative.

Testimonial

> I have had trouble on and off with my gallbladder for years. Sometimes I thought I was going to die. I used to take hot baths to help. All my friends said to have it removed, but I didn't like going that way. One day I saw Dr. Joe on TV talking about stem cells and activators. I called in and ordered three bottles [of] the GB. The doctor said it is good to go for three months so my bladder would get all the activators. So, I did. Well it didn't take three months. I was passing stones within a week and all my pain was gone. It has been almost a year and I have not had an attack since. I am so grateful.
>
> —BLANCH FROM NEW JERSEY

5. Chronic kidney disease and kidney failure

Kidneys are the body's filtration system, filtering the blood and ridding the body of toxic waste products such as urea from protein metabolism and uric acid. Kidneys also play a role in balancing our electrolyte levels (potassium and sodium) and our pH levels, controlling blood pressure, and stimulating red blood cell production.

When we get dehydrated from being out in the heat too long, from exercise, or from not properly hydrating throughout the day, the kidneys will hold or retain fluids until the urine is diluted enough to urinate.

---

* See my book *Bloodtypes, Bodytypes, and You* for more information.

Symptoms of chronic kidney disease and kidney failure

In the early stages of kidney disease you might have no symptoms at all, but if the condition becomes chronic and progresses to kidney failure, you might experience overall weakness, edema (water retention) that causes swelling in legs or feet, fatigue, shortness of breath, lethargy, and heart rhythm disturbances such as tachycardia (rapid heart rate), just to name a few of the symptoms.

Causes of chronic kidney disease and kidney failure

The causes of renal or kidney failure are vast. They can stem from medications to traumas, injuries, kidney stones, or infections such as sepsis.

Adult stem cell activators for chronic kidney disease and kidney failure

While conventional medicine prescribes various medications for kidney disease, again treating the symptoms, I like to visit the cellular biological levels to treat the root cause—damaged adult stem cells. As the kidney cells are repaired by the newly rejuvenated and repaired adult stem cells, the kidneys start to respond positively, as was the case with my ninety-two-year-old mother.

Just to witness personally how the progression of kidney failure in an elderly woman can be stopped by taking the adult stem cell activators is more than making these near miracle wonders evidence-based technology. In her case, she took the KDN activator for the kidneys.

Testimonial

> I began taking the KDN stem cell activator in November. My level was a 17. I went back to my doctor and my level is at 25!!! In one month. I will continue to take these forever!! I don't want to have to live on dialysis. This is an answer to prayer!! Thank you.
>
> —N. Cline from Georgia

> THANK YOU!! My husband's kidney output went up 10 percent with just one bottle!! His doctor was as excited as we were because he has been diagnosed with chronic kidney failure.
>
> —Mary from San Diego

Before moving on to the healthy lifestyle section of this book, let's review what we have learned so far. In section 1 we discovered that we all have been genetically blessed with our own natural cell repair crews—adult stem cells. We learned all about their efficacy and nearly miraculous abilities for repairing cells that have been damaged. When functioning properly, they keep our overall health and physiology in good working order.

We also explored how the advancements in stem cell technology and activation are the new disruptive therapies and treatments in regenerative medicine. We examined how they are replacing the old conventional medical approaches and procedures with new cutting-edge technologies by which you and I can opt for better and more effective ways of healing and repairing our bodies with results that resemble the miraculous.

In section 2 we discovered that the aging process, environmental toxicities, diseases, illnesses, and even traumas can cause our adult stem cells to lose their capacity to communicate properly from one cell to the other. Consequently, when our cells are damaged, they cannot perform properly and the affected organ or bodily system becomes problematic. Therefore, adult stem cell activation is vitally important to cellular health and performance.

The adult stem cells' inability to perform efficiently is manifested in the body as nagging degenerative health issues that seemingly never go away; horrific, constantly painful joints that ruin one's day-to-day routine; plus the emotional stress of living with the constant fear of degenerative diseases like diabetes, kidney failure, multiple sclerosis, and COPD.

Now in saying all that, I must tell you that you have two basic choices when it comes to managing your health—be proactive, or be reactive! As a doctor once said to me, "You can see me now or you can see me later!" My perspective is, if I do all I can to maintain optimum health, I may not have to see the doc, period!

As I said earlier in this book, I believe faithful caretaking of our bodies and health is not an option but an obligation. You and I have been created in such a way that our bodies require regular physical activity, proper nourishment, hydration, and detoxification. To optimize your health and quality of life, it is imperative to make healthy lifestyle practices an integral part of your lifestyle.

In the final section of this book I will provide you with some basic healthy lifestyle practices for making your body more energetic, more resilient against illness and disease, and more able to quickly recover should trauma hit. Regardless of what type of treatment or therapy you select—be it conventional medicine, alternative medicine, or naturopathic—healthy lifestyle practices will make all the difference. As a preventative measure or practice, a healthy, fit body will support your therapy and treatments and determine how well you bounce back from ill health or surgery and how well you repair and recover from injuries and physical trauma.

SECTION III

Healthy Living

I N THE PREVIOUS sections of this book you learned about being *reactive*. You learned all about the disruptive technologies and therapies in regenerative medicine regarding our adult stem cells and how they can miraculously heal and restore damaged joint tissues, correct or improve degenerative illnesses, and fortify cells for healthy longevity. Those treatments and therapies are necessary to correct health problems, which means that an individual is already in a poor state of health and has to be reactive!

But in this section we are going to be *proactive*!

We will look at a few areas central to healthy living. Our goal is to prepare the body to be more resilient, more energetic, and more vibrant. The idea behind healthy living is to be best prepared for what may come your way while enjoying the journey to its fullest. To do so you must be proactive.

Being proactive has many benefits and rewards, but it comes one day at a time. As you adapt to making healthy practices a part of your life, your life in turn will naturally respond positively, as it was designed to do.

I realize the topic of healthy living encompasses some broad topics, but before we delve into them, I want to take into consideration the mental and attitudinal connection to living a healthy life.

CHAPTER 7

THE RIGHT ATTITUDE
FOR CHANGE

THE INFORMATION FOUND in this section is intended to equip you with practical insights you may or may not have known at this point in your journey. They are necessary for you to implement if you want to be successful at obtaining a healthier, disease-free life and living that life to its fullest.

It all starts with the right mental attitude, which really makes the difference between success and failure. Having a great idea or goal is one thing, but having the correct mental attitude to make it come to fruition is another story. It is going to take the right mental attitude to make the changes necessary to accomplish your goals and desires. The correct attitude for success is an intangible and invisible commodity you possess, an invaluable asset that will make itself apparent to those around you—and to yourself—as you develop it.

All the insights, strategies, and methodologies in the world can't help you until you are ready to change. So, are you ready to make the changes necessary? I hope so. Just remember that you possess the power of the mind that will transform your present attitude toward your future health. This will be yours with only one condition and that is: change. Are you willing to change?

---

*The correct attitude for success is an
intangible and invisible commodity you
possess, an invaluable asset that will
make itself apparent to those around you—
and to yourself—as you develop it.*

ARE YOU WILLING TO CHANGE?

Because we humans are creatures of habit, change comes very hard. We have a tendency to gravitate to doing the same things over and over, sort of like burrowing ourselves in our own comfort zones.

As you think about the battle with keeping a healthy weight or the quality of health you desire, somewhere at some time you are going to need to make some changes in your lifestyle—if not for any other reason but for aging reasons alone. That's if you expect to live into those ripe old years with good health and quality of life. But you are going to need to make changes. It will be your decision whether they come by volunteering to change or by force.

No one is going to put a gun to your head if you don't volunteer to change. However, if you procrastinate long enough, it will be your health that forces you to make a change—if it isn't too late.

I have counseled many clients who told me they "knew" they needed to change their eating habits and make healthier lifestyle changes—*but*! For example, they would say, "I know I need to do something about exercising—*but*..." I don't which person is worse off, the one who isn't aware of their health or weight problem or the one who says they know they should change—*but*!

This mental attitude is partly a carryover of a crisis mentality that suggests, "If something isn't broken, why fix it?" Maintaining a healthy life or healthy weight for the long term doesn't stem from this kind of "fix-it-up-job" mentality but rather from an intelligent, preventative, ongoing perspective.

My hope for you is that you will volunteer to change.

Change can be a difficult thing for humankind because we are creatures of habit. People tend to repeat the same things over and over, even if what they are doing is not good for them or prevents them from improving their quality of life. Unfortunately, most of us have grown into adulthood without being taught the importance of the willingness to make changes.

Developing the attitude to change or the willingness to change must be ingrained in our minds from early in our lives. Regardless of what you're dealing with—be it maximizing your health, maintaining a healthy weight, or enjoying a good quality of life—unless you are willing to change, it will be impossible to reach your potential in any area of your life. So, when should we begin? I say as early in life as possible; and if you are older, then the time is *now!*

Willingness to change is absolutely the key to accomplishing your goals and dreams and to reaching your destiny in life. I ask again, are you willing to change? Change for the good! Change for the good of those you love.

MOTIVATION

You are in control of your health, weight, quality of life, and destiny—only you! To bring change—lasting change—into your life, you need motivation. Motivation is something everyone needs in order to make it to the end. When you identify motivational reasons for changing, it will be easier for you to make them happen.

Check out the following reasons to change. See if any of these reasons can help motivate you to make the changes in your life necessary to accomplish your goals.

- Family relationships: The dearest of all people need your example. They need you to be at your best! You need to be at your best for them! Change for the good!

- Friend relationships: Be an inspiration and encouragement to them. Show your friends you appreciate them by example. Change for the good!

- Health: Whether the goal is quality of life, losing weight, having more energy, or enjoying a pain-free, disease-free lifestyle, change for the good!

- Personal: Everyone deserves to look their best and feel good. And we all need to feel good about ourselves. Change for the good!

- Your future: If an ounce of prevention is worth a pound of cure, then a *pound* of prevention means you'll have *nothing* to cure! Change for the good!

OVERCOMING THE OBSTACLES

Deep down in your psyche there is a battle that rages. In fact, it has been raging for most of your life. Though its existence is usually ignored and subtle, it is extremely potent. If you aren't aware of this inner competition going on, you may never discover how to overcome the obstacles that present themselves at the moment of decision. These two opposing forces are vying for top position in your psyche. (Please note that I am not referring to making moral or immoral decisions.) Think of them as two voices inside your head: a "yes" voice and a "no" voice.

One voice is well developed. It's the play caller or the dominating voice you have learned to obey. The other is the lesser of the two voices and needs some personal training and deliberate attention.

Both voices are developed through years of input into your subconscious mind. And since the subconscious mind makes no distinction between positive affirmation and negative input, that which is most abundantly received will influence almost every decision you encounter, especially obstacles or challenges that present themselves.

Most of us deal with dominant "no" voices and weak, undeveloped "yes" voices because most of us have received more negative input than positive from our caretakers (possibly unintentionally) as well as other people and influences. Consequently, most people must work at being positive and confident in overcoming obstacles and challenges and attaining goals.

You might have heard the old computer science phrase, "garbage in, garbage out," which means that a computer's output can only be as accurate as the information entered into it. It is a principle that applies here. What goes into your subconscious mind will come out of your subconscious mind and influence your conscious mind. This happens regardless of whether you have received positive or negative input.

Your subconscious mind is like a psyche library that has filed away all negative and positive input throughout your life. Those stored negative and positive experiences influence your words, thoughts, self-worth, self-esteem, and level of confidence to overcome obstacles or challenges.

Like everyone else, you've stored up a litany of negative input from your caretakers, experiences, and life in general, whether you consciously remember it or not. As your subconscious mind filled with negative input, the "no" voice developed. Because you likely experienced less positive input, the "yes" voice developed much more slowly, or it hardly developed at all.

That's why, years later, you can find yourself afraid to make decisions, or find it difficult to stick with them because the "no" voice—being the loud play caller it is—has negatively influenced your decision-making process. For this reason, you might back down from challenging situations or might avoid attempting to attain significant goals or lifelong dreams. The control of the "no" voice prevents you and me from being all that we can be. It's time to stop listening to that voice!

AVOID NEGATIVE PEOPLE

It's easy to detect individuals who are controlled by the "no" voice because they are negative people. Their vocabulary consists of clichés such as "I can't," "Not me," "What if," "I doubt it," "Never happen," "I don't think so," "I'm afraid to," "I'm not good enough," and "I don't believe."

I'm sure you know one or two of these types; my suggestion is, stay as far away from these individuals as possible. They will only bring you down, dampen your aspirations, and get you out of focus.

Can you imagine raising a child and using those kinds of words all the time? Could you expect anything positive to come from that child's life? Do you think those negative seeds sown into their life would produce any positive fruit at all?

AH, THE "YES" VOICE

This voice proceeds from your subconscious mind like its negative counterpart, but its inventory is not as vast. For the most part, our caretakers were not big on pouring positive affirmations into our minds when rearing us. Consequently, its vocabulary has been reduced to only a few positive words that need expanding, and the volume certainly needs to be cranked up a little too.

The battle between these two opposites continues to rage. It is always going to be that way, but you can make a deliberate decision to invoke the "yes" voice. That's when your life will begin to change for the good.

That's when no matter how challenging the situation is, you'll hear a voice that says, "Yes, go for it!"

It only takes a few simple steps to make your "yes" louder than your "no":

1. Believe in yourself, and you will develop a whole new attitude and ability to listen to the "yes" voice when life's challenges come your way.

2. Avoid negative people as best you can. Refute all negative words and influences around you. Block the power of the "no" voice.

3. Expose yourself to positive people. Receive all positive words and influences. Develop the "yes" voice.

When you invoke the "yes" voice, your view of life opens and its challenges become positive. The goals you set for yourself will become doable and more rewarding. You will have done more than just reach your goal; you will have learned how to overcome challenges and obstacles.

As you will learn, being willing to make changes is the foundation for developing a positive mental attitude. It is half the battle for reaching a healthier, more disease-free life. Now that you have a better grip on the importance of establishing a positive mental attitude as part of a healthy lifestyle, let's look at some factual and practical applications.

WEIGHT AND YOUR HEALTH

Body genetics

Are you looking for the perfect body? I hope not. Besides beauty being in the eyes of the beholder, your dilemma will be, "What is a perfect body?"

Each of us has a genetic potential we can reach based on our genetic characteristics. So your potential won't be the same as somebody else's. Your body type and whether you have a thin or heavy frame will make your results different from others, but you can still eat and exercise in order to get the best results for your individual genetic characteristics. For example, an endomorphic body (large-framed structure) can never be an ectomorphic body (a petite structure) because we are talking about bone structure, not muscle or fat tissue.

From a genetic perspective, your unique body type with its unique structural characteristics must be factored into your healthy living strategy. It will also affect your ability to manage a healthy weight one way or the other.

One body type—the ectomorph—will have difficulty gaining weight, so people with this body type tend to be underweight. Another body type—the mesomorph—metabolizes calories well, so people with this body type can manage weight quite easily. People with the third body type—the endomorph—have the capability to easily gain weight.

By understanding what you are working with—and in this case, your unique body type—you can be best prepared for choosing which exercise program will best suit you. (For complete information about body genetics, see my book *Bloodtypes, Bodytypes, and You* in the appendix.)

Body composition

The quality of our weight is something most weight management enthusiasts overlook or are not aware of. Instead of being overly concerned about the *quantity* (how much we weigh), our body composition tells us what the *quality* of our weight is. The nice thing is that we do have control over our body composition. It is just a matter of making it a part of our healthy living plan.

I like using the analogy of a scale weighing a person at 150 pounds. The dependency on a scale to determine your weight is ineffective, as the scale is a terrible monitoring device. There could be 150 pounds of bricks, potatoes, or a human body on the scale and it can't distinguish the difference. Consequently, you can look great at 150 pounds or terrible.

That's why the quality of your weight (body composition) is ultimately the best means to determine your physique and illness potential. You calculate your body composition by comparing the percentage of your body fat vs. your lean muscle tissue. After taking a body composition test,* you will know your percentages of fat and muscle. By comparing these two measurements, you will know what weight category

---

* For complete information about body composition tests, body types, genetic weaknesses and strengths, please see my book *Bloodtypes, Bodytypes, and You* in the appendix.

you fall into, which will be far more accurate than the numbers on the bathroom scale.

The more attentive you are to your weight quality (body composition), the more tuned in you will be to potential health problems. We know that as a person continues to gain weight and becomes obese, it increases their chances of experiencing heart problems, diabetes, high blood pressure, stroke, gallbladder disease, and cancer of the colon, prostate, and breast. Being overweight creates regenerative problems as well, such as degenerative disc disease, bone demineralization, chronic joint pain, and cellular toxicity.

PROTEIN AND YOUR HEALTH

If you've ever read a book or article on nutrition or diet, chances are you already understand that carbohydrates stimulate an insulin response in the body, which is why diabetics have to monitor their carbohydrate intake very carefully. Just as carbohydrates stimulate an insulin response, protein stimulates another hormone named glucagon. Functioning opposite of insulin, glucagon encourages the body to burn fats, stabilizes the blood sugar, strengthens the immune system, suppresses the appetite, and supports protein synthesis. Glucagon, when stimulated by protein, will cause the body to burn fat more readily, reduce hunger and cravings for sweets, and protect the immune system. It is responsible for aiding the body in maintaining lean weight (body composition).

Your body needs adequate amounts of protein daily. As a rule, you should ingest 1 gram of protein for every 2.2 pounds of body weight. If you exercise regularly and are very physically active, then I would recommend 1 to 1.5 or more grams of protein per 2.2 pounds of body weight.

To prevent a hypoglycemic event (low blood sugar), prevent diabetes, and stabilize your blood sugar levels from spiking and plummeting, make sure your meals and snacks favor protein over carbohydrates. A meal that has more protein calories than carbohydrate calories is an *anabolic* meal.

Whether a snack or meal, eating more protein than carbs creates *anabolic momentum*. Protein food types (most accurately, those based on your blood type) will cause your body to burn fat for energy, thereby stabilizing blood sugar levels and supplying the muscle tissues with the nutrition needed for repair and building. Selecting protein in each of your meals and snacks will also improve your digestive and immune systems and stimulate weight loss (if you are overweight).

HYDRATION AND YOUR HEALTH

Drinking enough water is critical to staying well, especially at the cellular level. Try drinking an eight-ounce glass of water every hour, if you are not used to it. Spike it with lemon or lime or drink sparkling water if that's what it takes to get you to do it. To find out the amount of water you should drink daily, calculate half of your body weight in pounds. That number is how many ounces of water you should drink daily. For example, if you weigh 200 pounds, you need 100 ounces of water a day.

Avoid sodas and fruit drinks, and avoid fruit juices made from concentrates. Also, drinks with caffeine will contribute to dehydration, so herbal teas, particularly green tea, are better choices than coffee.

HUNGER OR APPETITE?

Have you ever stared down the refrigerator shelves or scanned the pantry and nothing looked appetizing? Or have you sat down at work and suddenly your stomach was growling? Well, I just described the difference between appetite and hunger.

There are physiological indications to measure hunger: growling sounds in your tummy and low blood sugar levels. When your metabolism needs nourishment, those two events occur. But what about when nothing jumped off the shelves in the pantry after you stared them down for fifteen minutes? That, my friend, is what we call your appetite at work, coping with unsolved emotional issues.

The inclination to become fat or overweight is induced by lifestyles that are full of the wrong food selections, including an abundance of processed and fast foods. We'll talk about the role of exercise in burning calories later. But for now, remember these three points when it comes to eating:

1. Eat when hungry.

2. Stop when satisfied (not stuffed).

3. Don't eat when not hungry—appetite/emotional eating.

Food nourishes our bodies, not our minds or emotions. There is nothing on your plate that can meet your emotional needs. Regardless of how you feel, your emotions should not be allowed to cross over to your plate of food. To safeguard your healthy lifestyle choices, remember what we discussed about boundaries.

Simple Guidelines to Avoid Emotional Eating

- If you are anxious or tense, go for a walk or have a workout.

- If you are depressed, call a friend who will make you laugh.

- When you feel stressed, pray, meditate, or do some relaxation exercises.

- When you are angry, forgive.

- When you are sad or lonely, hug someone.

- When you are tired, get some sleep.

- Do not eat when you are experiencing any of these emotions!

- Remember: You are not what you think you are. But what you think, you are!

Let's move on to what I refer to as a nutritional base for establishing a healthier body and life. Until one has established a base from food types as their primary source of nutrition, obtaining a healthy lifestyle, correcting health issues, correcting weight problems, or developing a powerful immune system will be very difficult.

CHAPTER 8

THE NUTRITIONAL BASE—FOOD

O BVIOUSLY, IT IS wise to have the right mental outlook before you take on any endeavor. With your boundaries in place and self-control ready to keep you on point, let's look at food from a different perspective, a perspective that is not about dieting.

I'm sure I am preaching to the choir at times, but we must consider all the variables when it comes to maintaining a lifestyle that supports a healthy weight. There are emotions directly tied into how we eat, how much we eat, and what we eat. Of course, there are also social and cultural influences that can get us looking at ourselves—our worth and value—from a negative perspective because of the perfect body image that Hollywood casts.

I have chosen not to compare the various types of diet programs on the market today in this section. I'm sure you know or have tried at least one of them and have your unique experience.

The topic I want to address is establishing a nutritional base of the right foods, which is ground zero for your health. In other words, your health is dependent upon what you put in your mouth. Remember the old adage, "garbage in, garbage out" that I brought up in the last chapter? It was a popular phrase in the early days of computing, so only those of us who are "of a certain age" might remember it!

But with all kidding aside, no matter what your age, it's a simple truth that the outcome of your overall health is directly related to the types of food you regularly eat. It is what happens at the cellular level—at the surface of your red blood cells—when you eat various types of food that makes all the difference. Once you have a sound nutritional base in place, managing your weight, naturally detoxifying the body, eliminating diseases, and being more vibrant and energetic will be the natural by-product.

As we look further into this topic, I believe this understanding will help you establish the most accurate nutritional base for you personally. From there you can build a healthier, more vibrant, disease-free body— healthy living.

GENETIC VS. GENERIC APPROACH TO EATING

When it comes to eating, I like to say there's the *generic* approach (one size fits all) and the *genetic* approach (eating the best foods for your individual body and blood type). My goal here is to demonstrate why the genetic approach is most accurate for establishing your individual nutritional base.

As I mentioned at the start of this chapter, what we eat has a direct impact on our health and it all happens as cellular responses. We know that not everyone responds the same way to the same food types. To make this most accurate, we are going to examine genetic characteristics among the four blood types.

Given a scenario of all things being equal, let's imagine all four blood types (A, B, AB and O) sitting down and eating the same meal. Within minutes to an hour after eating, everyone is going to respond differently. One type will have an increased level of energy, where the other type might feel a little sluggish, lethargic, or even hypoglycemic. Another will feel bloated and have some gurgling taking place in their tummy, maybe even some GERD events; and yet another will feel unsatisfied and not fully nourished.

When it comes to eating, I like to say there's the generic *approach (one size fits all) and the* genetic *approach (eating the best foods for your individual body and blood type).*

The premise of making food selections compatible with your blood type is based on a biochemical response that occurs at the surface of the red blood cells. It is not an approach to eating food types that is based on whether a food type is healthy or not. When we factor in the importance of our cells and their functions—in this scenario, red blood cells—it becomes very clear that the *genetic* approach to food selection establishes the most accurate nutritional base.

For over twenty years I have been advocating the concept of making food selections for your blood type through my book *Bloodtypes, Bodytypes, and You* via television and radio interviews, Skype, webinars, and conferences. I personally adhere to this approach to eating and have overcome several health issues by doing so. Overall, I find it most in tune with my body and how it responds. If I ever select food types that are not compatible with my blood type chemistry, my body puts me into a food type rejection crisis. For me, choosing which foods to eat is never a matter of being good or bad, but rather, how many days a week do I want to feel lousy, or well? And I believe your experience will be the same.

Over the years I have heard from many, many people all over the world who share the positive results they've experienced after eating the foods most chemically compatible with their blood types. Some of the results have been life changing from the standpoint of awareness of why some foods work as medicine for healing and other food types act as poison. After learning what their blood type is and eating accordingly, some have reported losing weight without even trying. Many have stated that they feel more energetic and more vibrant, and their illness profiles are improving. If I hadn't personally experienced the same amazing results for all these years, I would have been the first to dump the idea.

As I mentioned, the food types we eat have everything to do with the outcome of our health. For some people, making the switch to foods that are compatible with their blood type chemistry was the difference between being confined to a wheelchair in crippling pain and discovering a whole new, pain-free life.

I want to share a couple of testimonials from people who have had wonderful results in making their lives healthier, pain-free, and more energetic and vibrant. First is a wonderful testimonial from a woman who experienced total relief from chronic pain and is now a living, walking example of the difference it made.

> *Choosing which foods to eat is never a matter*
> *of being good or bad, but rather, how many*
> *days a week do I want to feel lousy, or well?*

It is with much gratitude that I share my life-changing story with you.

The summer of 2009, I was shopping for a gift in a bookstore. Not being a reader, I had walked through the book section and a book jumped off the shelf into my hands. It was called *Bloodtypes, Bodytypes, and You* by Joseph Christiano, ND, CNC. As I was leafing through the book, I was wondering why we didn't hear more about this. While waiting in line to purchase the book, I actually sold it to the lady behind me and had to go back to get another one for me.

Once I got home, I noticed the "Avoid List" and thought at that time that it would be difficult to follow as I didn't want to give up the foods that I liked so much, not realizing that these foods were sending my body into chaos. I have the rarest of types, AB, and only 4 percent of people in the United States have it. In the fall of 2010, my doctor sent me to a neurologist because the pain in my body was so debilitating that something had to be done.

I had a serious lower back injury in 1962 and I was diagnosed with osteoarthritis in 1986, with the MRI tests reflecting this between every vertebra in my spine. The fall of 2010 was so difficult that two prescriptions from the neurologist and four Motrin did not cover the pain as I was working my craft shows as an artist and in my daily life in general.

My pain had reached the point that I was no longer able to get in and out of the bathtub, and I knew that if something didn't change, I was headed for a wheelchair and a nursing home. The pain was in my left hip, thigh, calf, and top of my foot. *Here is where things got exciting!* In January 2011, I decided to get the book out and get serious about it. *Within one month,* by avoiding the "Avoid Foods," *I was off all meds* and a major turning point had occurred. For months I waited for that pain to return. I couldn't believe *the pain was gone and has not returned since*!! There was such a contrast from seriously feeling bad to feeling great that I thought, how could this have happened so fast? But after following the book and learning to *enjoy* the "Beneficial and Neutral Foods," my body began healing itself.

For years I had been seeing a chiropractor for misalignment of the spine with my left hip always off to the left visually. That is over. My spine is straight. Other areas that I noticed had improved after eating for my blood type was that having had an incontinence problem for a few years, I realized recently that eating according to my blood type has also affected the muscle tone in my entire body. What a relief this has been. My skin feels better, and I also realized that I was no longer using eye drops due to dry eyes. To this day, I am in awe of the energy that has resulted from following this change in the foods that are for my blood type. I even sleep better and feel more rested. Having turned seventy on February 23, 2013, people don't believe it. Many people say I look like I am in my fifties. This book and the way I eat now is definitely a God-given miracle.

Of the one hundred twenty-five foods recommended to avoid, I was eating fifty-one of them. I started gradually and have avoided these foods most of the time. I have learned to enjoy the beneficial and neutral foods even more.

The better that I feel, the more passionate I have become in sharing this rewarding experience with anyone that shows an interest. It has been an incredible ride!!

My wish is that everyone could experience their healing and feel better like I have. I HIGHLY recommend getting this book and following it right away. I only wish I had followed it when I first bought the book instead of waiting for my condition to get worse.

Thank you, Dr. Joe, for changing my life and helping me be *pain-free*!!

—BARB FROM MICHIGAN

As I read her story, it thrilled my heart to know my book helped her beat the odds she was facing like a life full of debilitating pain and agony, potentially being confined to a wheelchair, and having to continually take dangerous pain medications. She beat these odds just by making the dietary change from her former food selections (foods contributing to her painful condition) to food selections that aligned with her blood type chemistry. As I write this it has been seven years since she changed her eating habits and Barb is still enjoying a healthier, more energetic, pain-free life

BLOOD TYPES AND CARDIOVASCULAR DISEASE

In 2012, two large, prospective cohort studies showed that people with blood types A, B, and AB were at greater risk of coronary heart disease (CHD) than people with type O, according to Lu Qi, PhD, of the Harvard School of Public Health, and colleagues. You can read more about their findings at http://www.everydayhealth.com /heart-health/0815/type-o-blood-carries-lower-heart-disease-risk.aspx and http://www.medpagetoday.com/MeetingCoverage/AHA/29804. The findings of these researchers are nearly 100 percent accurate with our findings and experience with the genetic characteristics of blood type ABO patients and cardiovascular disease.

In addition to these studies, in this chapter I will (1) provide additional information from my studies and experience in working with the ABO blood type groups, blood type nutrition (diet), and cardiovascular disease, including the unique genetic predispositions of each blood type, and (2) provide the "answer" to the blood type/cardiovascular dilemma that satisfies Dr. Lu Qi's uncertainty about the cause, with study chart and blood type characteristics.

BLOOD TYPES AND BLOOD VISCOSITY

A very significant reason for one blood type having a greater potential for experiencing premature cardiovascular disease than another is a difference in blood viscosity. Blood viscosity is determined by the ease or lack of ease with which blood flows through miles of arterial walls throughout the body. When the blood becomes sluggish or thick, it creates a propensity for cardiovascular disease. Certain blood types naturally have a more sluggish or thick blood viscosity than others. This blood type characteristic contributes to potential cardiovascular disease earlier in life. When diet goes unaddressed, the likelihood of blood cells clotting or clumping together is great.

This phenomenon varies among each blood type. For example:

- The O and B blood type individuals are genetically predisposed to have very thin blood viscosity, the O being the thinner of the two.

- The A and AB types have very thick or sticky blood viscosity.

Though the higher risk of CHD is part of the illness profile of the A and AB blood types, people of all blood types can be affected when eating foods that are incompatible with their blood type. The answer to this dilemma is found in following a blood type nutrition or diet. (See my book *Bloodtypes, Bodytypes, and You* for more information.) It is when this condition goes unchecked that premature heart disease occurs.

ALKALINE PHOSPHATE ENZYME SECRETIONS

Another genetic characteristic that differs among the various blood types and contributes to blood viscosity and the potential for premature cardiovascular disease is the level of intestinal alkaline phosphate enzyme secretions. These secretions naturally help break down long-chain fatty molecules in the blood. The higher the secretion levels, the better the body can break down these long chain fatty molecules. These secretions are the body's natural anti-cholesterol bombs that help fight elevated cholesterol and premature cardiovascular disease.

When we compare the four blood types—O, A, B, and AB—with the secretion levels of intestinal alkaline phosphate enzymes, we see a difference in this phenomenon. For example:

- The O blood type individual has high secretion levels.

- The B blood type individual has moderate secretion levels.

- The A blood type individual has very low secretion levels.

- The AB blood type individual has very low secretion levels.

By genetic predisposition, one blood type has an advantage over the others in fending off premature cardiovascular disease. When certain food types are allowed in the diet, they prohibit or disrupt the secretion of the intestinal alkaline phosphate enzymes, which leads to the potential for premature cardiovascular disease.

PEPTIC ACID VS. CARDIOVASCULAR DISEASE

Blood type nutrition or diet most significantly contributes to preventing and/or lessening the potential for developing cardiovascular disease. When diet is incorrect, the potential increases for other common diseases such as acid reflux, irritable bowel syndrome (IBS), stomach pain, and peptic ulcers to occur. The goal is to maintain the correct environment per blood type.

The blood type O individual secretes high levels of peptic acid in the stomach, providing the perfect digestive environment for breaking down dense proteins such as red meat, therefore enhancing proper digestion and assimilation. Similarly, the B blood type individual experiences the same characteristics but at a moderate secretion.

On the other hand, we have the A and AB blood type individuals, who have more of an alkaline environment with low peptic acid secretions in the stomach. This condition causes their digestive system to struggle with breaking down dense protein, causing stomach and colon distress. Colon toxicity builds up due to undigested food and not only lends to colon health issues like constipation, impacted fecal matter, and even colon cancer, but also contributes to their already thick or sluggish blood viscosity.

This chart below represents a study I was involved in that was based on 5,200 individuals and their blood type, gender, age, and various diseases. It was clear to see that certain blood types had the propensity for experiencing some of these diseases early in life while other blood types seemed to dodge the bullet and not experience them until later. Upon our analysis of the criteria (notwithstanding the possibility of other factors) it was our conclusion that the individual could greatly correct or eliminate their health issue by following a blood type nutrition plan or diet.

COMPOSITE GRAPHS PROFILING
MORTALITY STATISTICS BY DISEASE

Heart Disease (heart attack, heart failure, heart disease, etc.)

Age	Under 40		40-49		50-59		60-69		70-79		80-89		90-99		Over 100		Total
	M	F	M	F	M	F	M	F	M	F	M	F	M	F	M	F	
Type A	1.8	0.4	3.0		9.5	2.2	12.1	1.3	3.5	2.6		0.4	0.4				37.2%
Type B	0.9	0.9			0.9		0.9	0.9	4.6	5.6	1.8	3.7		0.9			21.1%
Type AB			0.4	0.4	0.4	0.4	12.7	0.4	10.6	6.3							31.6%
Type O								0.4	2.2	0.8	3.6	3.1	4.0	2.2		0.8	17.1%
TOTAL %	2.7	1.3	3.4	0.4	10.8	2.6	25.7	3.0	20.9	15.3	5.4	7.2	4.4	3.1		0.8	

Cancer

Age	Under 40		40-49		50-59		60-69		70-79		80-89		90-99		Over 100		Total
	M	F	M	F	M	F	M	F	M	F	M	F	M	F	M	F	
Type A	2.2	4.5	2.6	6.3	7.6	4.9	9.4	6.3	4.0	4.5	0.9	0.4					53.6%
Type B		1.8	0.9	2.8	0.9	0.9	4.6	1.8	4.6	3.7	3.7	1.8	0.9				28.4%
Type AB			4.2	10.6	4.2	2.1	14.8	4.2	6.3	2.1							48.5%
Type O				0.4	0.8	0.8	1.2	1.2	1.6	3.1	4.9	4.9	0.4	0.4			19.7%
TOTAL %	2.2	6.3	7.7	20.1	13.5	8.7	30.0	13.5	16.5	13.4	9.5	7.1	1.3	0.4			

Diabetes

Age	50-59		60-69		70-79		80-89		90-99		Over 100		Total
	M	F	M	F	M	F	M	F	M	F	M	F	
Type A		0.9		2.2	1.7	1.3							6.1%
Type B					2.8		1.8	1.8					6.4%
Type AB			0.8	0.4									1.2%
Type O					0.4	2.2	1.2	2.2					6.0%
TOTAL %		0.9	0.8	2.6	4.9	3.5	3.0	4.0					

Natural Causes

Age	50-59		60-69		70-79		80-89		90-99		Over 100		Total
	M	F	M	F	M	F	M	F	M	F	M	F	
Type A			0.4	0.4		0.8	0.4	0.4					2.4%
Type B					0.4		4.6	5.6	5.6	4.6			20.8%
Type AB					0.4		0.4	0.4					1.2%
Type O						0.4	4.9	3.1	10.3	9.4	3.6	1.2	32.9%
TOTAL %			0.4	0.4	0.8	1.2	10.3	9.5	15.9	14.0	3.6	1.2	

BLOOD TYPE NUTRITION VS. DISEASES

To support a healthy, disease-free, vibrant life, we must start with a solid nutritional base. In our studies and experience, it has been revealed that all of us have genetically predisposed characteristics associated with our blood type. One blood type may have favorable genetic characteristics to fend off diseases while another has unfavorable genetic characteristics that make them susceptible to diseases.

When considering the powerful role of our blood type with diet, everything changes. When we adhere to blood type nutrition (diet) as our nutritional base, we are better equipped to reduce and/or prevent premature health disorders and diseases such as cardiovascular disease. (For complete daily menus, meal planning, recipes, and comprehensive information per blood type and related material, please see my book *Bloodtypes, Bodytypes, and You* in the appendix.)

TESTIMONIAL

Ever since I was introduced to *Bloodtypes, Bodytypes, and You* by Dr. Joe in 2006, I hsave had the best health among my peers. When people ask what nutritional plan I'm pursuing, without hesitation I refer them to Dr. Joe's resources and incredible website. My wife and I have utilized this incredible information continuously, and now our children are following the plan. Their growth and development have been exceptional to say the least. Both our boys are in the 90th plus percentile in development with exceptional health, and we truly believe this life-changing information has radically changed our health for generations to come. We are indebted tso Dr. Joe's investment into our lives through his incredible resources. We are blessed beyond belief!

—RYAN AND ALEXANDRIA McCOLLISTER

CHAPTER 9

SUPPLEMENTS

WHEN I CONSIDER the concept of taking nutritional supplements, it's not an option. I see it as a necessary and invaluable complement to the nutrients I receive from my diet or food type sources. I'll use an analogy to make my point.

In an orchestra, there are many parts and players. Each musician has his or her unique instrument and talent, and together they contribute the tones, sounds, and pitches to benefit the other orchestra members. For example, there's the woodwind section, the string section, the horn section, and so on. Each musician has his or her own music stand with specific music to play. They all dress to the tee and collectively equip the orchestra for the makings of a magnificent musical piece—until they warm up and practice their instruments! Then there seems to be something missing: the *maestro*, the orchestra leader!

The maestro complements all the parts and players by pulling their talents together. Without the maestro, it would be impossible for the orchestra to accomplish its ultimate purpose of making harmonious music together.

So it is with nutritional supplements. They complement a person's nutrient uptake from the food types they consume. Without them, particularly when deficiencies occur, the body lacks the nutrients necessary for optimum functionality.

SUPPLEMENTS—BASIC AND SPECIFIC

Personally, I have been taking nutritional supplements for fifty years. It has been one of the mainstays of the healthy practices I've lived by. I recall taking forty beef liver tablets, thirty protein tablets, and olive oil every day when I was only sixteen years old.

Today, if you were in my house and peeked into the pantry, you would see an assortment of bottles with capsules, liquid drops, and sprays that I take daily. I have a philosophy about the benefits of taking nutritional supplements: they enable me to be *basic* and *specific* regarding which nutrient(s) I require at a specific time. Let me explain what I mean.

As a simple *basic* approach, I strongly recommend taking a good daily multiple vitamin and mineral supplement. This basic approach covers most of the bases regarding daily nutritional demands. A daily dose of multiple vitamins and minerals is the perfect complement to one who is looking for the addition nutrients they are not getting from their diet. It's a means of fortifying their overall daily nutrient intake.

This builds another layer onto the nutritional base I covered in chapter 8. In addition to choosing the right types of foods, it's important to understand that their *bioavailability*—the degree to which their nutrients are absorbed into your body—may not be optimal. That's why supplementing the *basic* vitamins and minerals your body needs is important.

I have a philosophy about the benefits of taking nutritional supplements: they enable me to be basic *and* specific *regarding which nutrient(s) I require at a specific time.*

Another benefit of supplementing is the ability to be *specific*. As your physical demands increase—whether you're combatting an illness, you've started to exercise or participate in sports, or you're dealing with chronic pain or some degenerative disease—it is important to adjust your nutrient uptake to meet these *specific* new demands. In the same way I've talked about targeting the stem cell activators to address specific health conditions, you can target your supplements in ways that complement these stem cell activators and enhance their effectiveness.

Here is a simple example of how I customize my own nutritional supplements to meet my specific needs. Because I deal quite a bit with inflammation in my shoulder and lower back, I take specific supplements to complement the adult stem cell activator for connective tissue.

When I sense the need (I start to feel the pain caused by the inflammation), I will up my daily dose of sockeye salmon oil from Alaska, turmeric with peprine, and a multiple enzyme supplement with serrapeptase. The combination of these nutritional supplements does wonders to reduce the effects of inflammation in my joints, ligaments, and arteries.

Before we go on, I need to make one thing perfectly clear. You can't eat whatever you want and then take a multivitamin or other supplement and think it makes up for the lack of nutrition in your poor eating habits. Most supplements are basically useless if you are not making food selections for your blood type. The supplements are not the nutritional base; your food is. Without that foundation, the supplements have nothing to build upon.

When I eat foods that are not compatible with my blood type, within only a few days I notice my joints, back, and neck all start feeling painful from inflammation. So it is vitally important to keep that food type base in place before selecting supplements.

Health Benefits of Apple Cider Vinegar

There are other natural means for improving and correcting health problems along with taking supplements. One natural remedy is apple cider vinegar. If you've ever looked it up online, you know the list of health benefits from this seemingly ordinary product is practically endless. For example, if you are experiencing bloating, indigestion, stomach discomfort, or even GERD, here is something I find works for me every time.

First thing after rising from bed, I drink a 12-ounce glass of water with 2 tablespoons of Bragg's apple cider vinegar and ½ teaspoon of baking soda. This combination (another option is to take them independent of each other) is great for balancing your stomach pH. Most of the time when a person is hurting from acid reflux or acidic stomach, they are recommended to take "the purple pill"—the very thing you should not take, in my opinion. When you experience the effects of acid discomfort, it generally means *you do not have enough* stomach acid, not the opposite. Once you balance your pH, all the symptoms should disappear.

Another thing you may find helpful is to take apple cider vinegar three times throughout the day mixed in water. If the taste is too pungent, then add some local honey to your drink. You can even make a huge pitcher full of water, apple cider vinegar, and honey and keep it refrigerated for up to a week. When we were young my mother would make this every day for us—we called it bug juice!

In my opinion, the only apple cider vinegar that provides the multiple health benefits I've referred to is Bragg's. Google it and you can read all about it!

One last tip for acid discomfort in the stomach, esophagus, or throat: try eating slices of fresh ginger when your symptoms flare up. In the past I have taken two or three slices of ginger and chewed on them, and within a half hour or so, all the acid discomfort was gone. This is great for reducing the inflammation and healing the sensitive tissue. (If you do this and then eat accurately for your blood type, you shouldn't experience any future acid issues.)

BASIC AND SPECIFIC SUPPLEMENTS TO CONSIDER*

Just to make things simple, this list is far from being exhaustive. I want to give you some basic and specific supplement suggestions. As you become more tuned in to your body and how it responds, when greater demands appear, you will know what you need to take to heal and restore your body back to natural health. If you have health conditions or are taking medications, be sure to consult your doctor before changing or supplementing your diet.

Other than grouping them into basic and specific categories, these supplements are not listed in any particular order.

Basics

- AM/PM MULTIVITAMINS—this multiple vitamin and mineral supplement covers all the bases for general well-being and complementing the nutrient uptake from the food types you ingest.

- B-VITAMIN COMPLEX (for women)—this supplement has all the members of the B-vitamin family that will help meet the nutritional requirements of women.

---

* Note: For more information about these and more supplements, go to www.bodyredesigning.com or call 1-800-259-2639.

- CONCENTRACE (liquid trace minerals)—this supplement helps correct bunions, elevated uric acid–related disorders, and more. Our bodies do not produce trace minerals, and approximately seventy-two of them are not found in our food sources or soil either. Therefore, most people are trace mineral deficient and will greatly benefit from supplementing them daily.

Specifics

- PROST-EZE (prostate support for men)—this supplement provides vitally important nutrients for a healthy functioning prostate. A nourished prostate is a healthier prostate. Supplementing specifically for the prostate is a preventive measure to help avoid the onset of prostate cancer.

- COOLED OFF—this supplement has specific anti-inflammatory nutrients for counterpunching the negative, painful effects of inflamed joints, muscles, and soft tissue.

- TURMERIC 750mg—this supplement has specific anti-inflammatory nutrients for counterpunching the negative, painful effects of inflamed joints, muscles, and soft tissue.

- IMMUNE SUPPORT—this supplement boosts the body's defense system for combating germs, infections, diseases, viruses, bacteria, and more.

- HGH SUPPORT (bioengineered hormone support)—this supplement provides the body with nutrients specific for our own natural hormonal secretion of HGH and is vitally important for a litany of antiaging reasons.

- WOMAN'S SUPPORT—this supplement provides specific nutrients for a woman's unique hormonal requirements, making it essential for optimal health and vibrancy.

- TRIM (weight loss)—this caffeine-free amino acid combo works to burn fat and boost metabolism.

- DIGESTIVE COMPLEX (digestive support)—after the age of thirty, most of us lose the ability to produce ample enzyme secretion in our stomachs. As we age, stomach and digestive disorders are common but shouldn't be. The root cause is the lack of enzymatic action or digestion enzyme secretion.

As I mentioned above, this list of supplements is an example of a few very important supplements. Daily nutritional supplementation goes a long, long way to help you achieve a healthy lifestyle—it has for me. Learning more about how your body functions—and what it requires to function as it did when you were younger—will help you make these lifestyle changes easier.

As you put these healthy habits into practice, your entire life will take on a whole new level of wellness and you will start to appreciate how wonderfully your body has been fashioned. Then your hope for a healthier and more youthful life as you get older will become a reality.

Whether you are struggling with chronic pain, recent injuries, overall weakness, or disease, please know that your body was designed to heal itself. Instead of following the conventional medical methods of treating your symptoms as the first line of defense, I hope that you will give your body the benefit of the doubt and test everything naturally first!

I encourage you to totally exhaust every natural alternative protocol, nutritional supplement, treatment, and remedy that's available to you. Allow natural health to be your first line of defense for eradicating the root cause(s) of your symptoms, pain, and poor health conditions. Only when all else has failed may you have no choice but to seek conventional medicine and its approach to dealing with your symptoms.

Our Creator didn't forget a thing when He designed these bodies of ours. He is the giver of eternal and physical life, and it is our responsibility to take control of our lives and do the things that will support, build up, and strengthen our bodies. No one else can do it for us.

As you step out and make healthy lifestyle changes, remember it won't be one orchestra member that makes the difference but rather the entire orchestra working in harmony together to accomplish the mission.

CHAPTER 10

ANTIAGING

S OME OF YOU reading this book are probably baby boomers—Americans born between 1946 and 1964. It is common knowledge that people in your parents' generation, the pre-boomer generation, are now living past their midnineties and into their hundreds—imagine that! And if this trend continues as projected, what are you and I doing today to support a greater quality of life for the next twenty, thirty, or forty years to come?

I find this antiaging mind-set very fascinating for a couple of reasons. First, I see an overemphasis placed on getting old in general. Many are worried about the lines and wrinkles on their faces, the double chins, and the graying or receding of the hair. I think too much thinking goes into looking younger. Second, I simply believe that when a person works at living a healthy lifestyle and is consistent at it, they will naturally develop a younger, more youthful appearance. As I age, I try to aim toward looking *healthy* rather than looking *young*. Again, it is not all about our looks but our bodily functions that keep us looking healthy.

I imagine you are like everyone else who has their reason to be concerned about aging and what to do to slow it down. Are you afraid of the inevitable or are you freaking out because the mirror on the wall doesn't seem to line up with the way you perceive yourself?

Recently I had my fiftieth-year high school class reunion but couldn't attend it. So a good friend of mine told me all about it and how our classmates looked these days. One topic he mentioned to me that I found to be sort of an eye-opener was what he noticed in the main room of the facility where the dance floor was. He said all the classmates and their spouses were having a good time dancing, but as they walked off the dance floor, he could see some of them had a limp, some moved slower than others, and stiff lower backs causing them to walk bent over were obvious. I thought to myself, "Well bless their hearts for at least getting out there and moving around to have fun."

He said some couldn't or didn't dance because they had walkers or canes, and one was in a wheelchair, and the rest were somewhere in between. Of course, some of the jocks, the low percentage of my former classmates, moved around well and looked healthy and youthful for their age. As I learned from my friend, those classmates stay very active. He also sent me photos, and as I looked at them, I thought to myself, "It wasn't the excess weight, gray hair, receding hair lines, or bald heads that stood out and made me think of the aging factor."

Understanding the difference between chronological age and functional age and what to do about it puts you on the right track to slow the aging process.

Though everyone was nearly the same age, give or take a year or two, what really stood out to me as my friend shared with me was the huge gap between the few who could move around the entire day and those who struggled. You know what I mean, the difference in chronological age and functional age. It was quite an eye-opener, as I said, and reminds me to keep being physically active, keep a positive attitude, and enjoy my life!

I realize life does not come with any guarantees (except death and taxes, as the saying goes), but I can guarantee there is a way that you can enjoy a greater quality of life for as long as you live. The battle with aging encompasses every area of life, but understanding the difference between chronological age and functional age and what to do about it puts you on the right track to slow the aging process.

CHRONOLOGICAL AGE VS. FUNCTIONAL AGE

One of the worst things a person can do as they age is become less physically active. Do you find yourself parking closer to the store so you don't have to walk as far? Do you sit more than you move around the office or your house? If you are not careful, you will adapt a sedentary lifestyle, and before you know it, your functional age will surpass your chronological age. This commonly happens as we age, but there are things that can be done.

I'm certain you could use more energy, would like to recover quicker from sickness or injuries, and even sleep better. We will discuss these benefits later in this section, but right now let's look at this rivalry between our age and how well we perform our daily activities.

With regards to antiaging and ensuring a better quality of life, the true battle lies between chronological age and functional age. In other words, changing our chronological age is obviously impossible. That's a no brainer! But our functional age is an entirely different story. Not only can it be improved upon, but it can enhance a more vibrant life.

Sitting Is the New Smoking

I encourage you to read the eye-opening blog post written by Diana Gerstacker and posted at www.huffingtonpost.com. It's called "Sitting Is the New Smoking: Ways a Sedentary Lifestyle Is Killing You." [1] It references a *Los Angeles Times* interview with Dr. James Levine, director of the Mayo Clinic-Arizona State University Obesity Solutions Initiative. It quotes Dr. Levine as summing up his research findings about our increasingly sedentary lifestyles in the following way: "Sitting is more dangerous than smoking, kills more people than HIV and is more treacherous than parachuting. We are sitting ourselves to death." [2]

Unintentionally, many people who work long hours at the computer or sitting at their desks are creating worsened conditions for their joints, ligaments, and muscles, not to mention lack of blood circulation, muscle stimulation, and future musculoskeletal problems. Poor posture like slumping over the keyboard places undue stress on the cervical joints in the neck, places pressure on nerves, and creates nerve pain and dysfunction. Muscles are shortened while opposite muscles are overstretched. The list goes on and on. Until one makes an all-out effort to compensate for the sedentary lifestyle, premature ill-health conditions will be expected.

As the sidebar on the previous page illustrates, living a sedentary lifestyle puts your health in a downward spiral, which in turn increases deterioration of the body, reduces the things you can do pain-free, and eventually induces premature death. Doesn't sound so good, does it?

The question that begs to be asked is, are our bodies slowing down because of age or are there essential elements to our physiology causing the slowdown?

On the other hand, if we take the proper measures to strengthen our bodies with regular exercise, nourish our bodies with food selections for our blood type, stay properly hydrated, add nutritional supplements for additional nutrients, address our hormone levels, and keep a positive mental attitude, we just might function like a person ten, fifteen, or twenty years younger with fewer illnesses and less pain.

So, the question that begs to be asked is, are our bodies slowing down because of age or are there essential elements to our physiology causing the slowdown?

The physical and mental conditions of the elderly at an assisted living facility can be quite depressing. But from a positive perspective, it can be very motivating to do something now to slow down that aging process.

Senior Functional Classifications

Here is list of classifications of the senior population that depicts the general digression and decline in health, activity levels, and quality of life. What you do about it is up to you.

- **Physically Elite**. This group represents a very small percentage of seniors. They train daily and compete in sports such as the Senior Olympics or triathlons, or they participate regularly in vigorous activities or group fitness classes. These seniors can participate in high-risk activities such as weightlifting and usually perform at the highest level.

- **Physically Fit**. This is a larger group than the elite group, but it is still a small percentage of the population. These seniors typically participate in exercise sessions at least two times per week. They venture out and do some rollerblading or play tennis. They can participate in endurance sports like power walking, and they are at low risk for falling into the "physically frail" category.

- **Physically Independent**. This group of seniors shows signs of loss in balance, coordination, strength, and flexibility. They are the largest group of seniors and range from minimally active to somewhat functionally independent. They may engage in crafts or gardening and perhaps take light walks. They participate in low-level activities such as playing golf. They don't show any debilitating symptoms, but an injury or illness could affect their mobility and physical function. They are apt to fall into the "physically frail" category.

- **Physically Frail**. These seniors perform daily activities that are not very demanding, such as shopping and cleaning. They are capable of light activities but usually sit around and watch television. In many cases, they just stay at home.

- **Physically Dependent**. This group represents a small percentage of seniors who are often in wheelchairs and need home care. Basically, they spend much of their money on health care.

- **Totally Disabled**. This small group of seniors cannot stand or walk. They must rely on complete assistance from a professional health-care staff.

Let's look at how regular exercise impacts your functional age.

EXERCISE AND FUNCTIONAL AGE

As you review the classifications in the sidebar above, it is easy to see the parallels. As aging men and women decline in daily activities, they also decline in physical condition. Does the chronological age factor determine activity level, or is the functional age determined by the activity involvement?

I realize nobody wants to talk about or even think about the fact that they are getting older. Of course, it doesn't help to see the ultra-thin Hollywood celebrities that our society throws in our faces either. It can be intimidating and depressing if we allow those younger generations to influence our minds. They are younger and they should be in good shape.

What about the rest of us who are older than that younger generation and are dealing with the aging process and the way our bodies act and react lately? Those Hollywood bodies may be a younger generation strutting their stuff right now, but not so long from now they will also face the perils of getting older.

You are as old as you are (you can't change your age), but you can do something about your physical fitness condition at your age. The older you get, the more important it becomes for you to exercise.

Many of us think the aging process doesn't begin until we reach our parents' age, but the fact of the matter is, the aging process begins immediately after birth. Often we are unaware of the aging process until we hit our forties, which is when many of the antiaging hormones drop off significantly.

As we age, our bodies become more fragile because activity levels decrease. We sit more and move less, and our bones deteriorate through demineralization. This sedentary lifestyle with its lack of physical activity contributes to the dysfunction and ill health of the joints, and day-to-day life in general becomes a burden. This condition is compounded by a loss of muscle tissue (called muscle atrophy) because of physical inactivity. Consequently, everyday tasks become a task. Physical inactivity is the nemesis of a successful weight loss and weight management lifestyle. On top of that, it messes with our mental attitude—and we all know the importance of maintaining the right attitude, don't we?

And if that isn't enough, there are other factors such as our genetic individuality/heredity, gender, physical injuries, and overall lifestyle practices that need to be considered. Then finally throw in a litany of premature chronic diseases and you have just raised your "functional age."

---

*It's not what age you are, but
what you do with what you have!*

Functional age is based on your physical fitness condition. The lower your functional age, the better. Lowering your functional age must become your constant goal, and it is determined by your ability to physically function at a younger age than your actual chronological age. If you are actively involved in regular exercise, you will reduce your functional age; on the contrary, by living a sedentary lifestyle, you will heighten your functional age.

For example, if you are a forty-five-year-old and do not exercise and your physical fitness condition is poor, I guarantee you probably feel and move like a sixty-year-old person rather than the forty-five-year-old person you are. Or if you are a sixty-year-old who exercises regularly and is in good physical fitness condition, you may very well function as a thirty-year-old individual. Remember, your functional age is determined by other factors such as genetics and environmental adaptations, but exercise plays a huge role in it.

So what's the big deal about getting older anyway? It's not what age you are, but what you do with what you have! Well, start doing something about it and exercise regularly.

Things to Consider

To better prepare yourself, read through the following considerations as you form your plan to take the road that leads you to being healthier and more physically fit.

- See a doctor before beginning your exercise program, especially if you are over thirty-five and have been inactive for several years. It's good to have a bird's-eye view of what is going on inside and the assurance of a health-care professional.

- Factor in your age before jumping into any exercise program. I have worked with many men and women in their midthirties who nearly bought the farm because they forgot they weren't that spring chicken anymore. Consider your age, current activity level, and overall fitness condition beforehand.

- How long has it been since you trained with free weights or exercise equipment on a regular basis? Are you making a comeback, or are you a beginner? Don't expect to reach your goals in one workout.

Regardless of your exercise background, your long-term success must start off one step at a time.

- Are you interested in getting in shape to assist your athletic ability and performance? If so, then your training program must be designed for sports or be sports specific.

- Are you a female with specific goals like losing a certain amount of weight so you can wear those clothes that have been hanging in your closet since you were a couple sizes smaller? Then your exercise protocol must be designed to accommodate and assist in body fat reduction.

- Are you lacking energy, strength, or balance in your physique? Again, these areas of concern and interest must be factored into your exercise strategy before you start. Should the program place the emphasis on cardiovascular conditioning or strength training and body redesigning?

- What are your body's genetic limitations? Do you know how to troubleshoot your genetic problem areas? Your program must be tailored to your body's genetic specifics or you will be spinning your wheels and results will come very, very slowly.

- Have fun with exercise. Your regular program should be designed to meet your specific goals, but be sure to stay physically active in addition to your program.

- Be sure to throw in some physical activities outside the gym, such as tennis, volleyball, golf, or any other sport or activity that will keep the blood flowing.

Staying physically active is key to high energy, less body fat, better appearance, less illness, healthy longevity, and a host of other benefits. Therefore, take the time to apply the previous information to your lifestyle.

HORMONES AND YOUR HEALTH

I know you have heard that as we age, we start experiencing age-related symptoms like sagging skin, thinning and graying hair, hot flashes, less muscle tissue, pot bellies, extra body fat, weakness, painful joints, terrible digestive pain, and less energy. But did you know that those symptoms or conditions *are not from aging but rather from less hormone secretion?*

If you are over thirty years of age, then your hormonal secretion levels are significantly diminishing, less effective, and less usable to sustain your once-youthful health. This downward spiral will continue over the years to come *if you don't do something about it now!*

Below I have an abbreviated list of questions and answers that target the aging process and the role hormones play in the war against aging. Let's look at the cause and effect of hormone secretion or lack thereof and some antiaging measures we can take as we enter our midthirties, midlife, senior years, and older ages.

Q1: Why are hormones still important as we age?

A: Hormones are essential to every cell in our body, and that's huge when you consider we are made up of trillions and trillions of cells. Normal hormonal levels translate to healthy cells, which are directly related to healthy bodily functions. Hormones assist the body with energy, muscle recovery (from work, exercise, or surgeries), sleep, mental awareness, and mental cognizance. Hormones are necessary for healthy skin and organ/gland function. Normal hormone levels slow down declining health and can reverse it by enhancing the body's recuperative powers.

Q2: Do sex hormones—testosterone and estrogen—decline as people age? Is there any reason to be concerned with these hormones after the age of forty-five, fifty, sixty, and older, or should we just let 'em go (who cares)?

A: Men and women should be concerned about managing their hormonal levels if they are interested in optimum physical and emotional health. Raising our sex hormones to physiological levels restores and enhances that intimate part of life that is lost over time. We can take a variety of medications for erectile dysfunction (ED) or problems with libido, but not without serious side effects. We can only expect to enjoy a vibrant, sexually active life well into our twilight years by correcting our hormonal deficiencies naturally with certain nutritional supplementation and stem cell activation.

Q3: What is the most important hormone for antiaging?

A: Human growth hormone is key and responsible for normalizing and correcting bodily functions such as reducing PMS symptoms and hot flashes/menopause (women) and andropause (men), improving immune system function, improving cardiac and lung function, reducing body fat, increasing muscle mass, increasing libido and sexual performance, increasing bone density, lessening the risk of osteoporosis, reducing the onset of type 2 diabetes, thickening hair, and much more.

Q4: Do environmental toxins contribute to hormone imbalance? And if so, which ones are the worst culprits?

A: Our cells and tissues are damaged by environmental toxins and pollutants plus oxidative damage by free radicals. Superoxides, hydroxyl radicals, peroxides, and hydroperoxides are examples of free radicals. This damage occurs by inhaling environmental toxins such as the gaseous emissions from automobiles, buses, and trucks. (Illness, disease, medication, poor food selection, poor digestion, lack of exercise, stress, and a weakened immune system also contribute to cellular damage.) Environmental pollutants include dangerous pesticides like Roundup, which contains a component of Agent Orange and is one of the worst.[3]

Many individuals suffer from pain and illnesses caused by impaired and unbalanced molecules. These impaired molecules attach themselves to healthy cells in the body. Wherever they attach themselves, they cause a rapid oxidation process, which results in cell damage and the development of health problems. For example, if there is free radical damage to the cells in the walls of the arteries, then plaque buildup is eminent. If cellular damage occurs in the joints, then inflammation and arthritic pain and discomfort are experienced.

One of the most common (but undetected by the medical community) root causes of many diseases and premature aging factors is petroleum by-products or junk estrogens. These toxic materials are responsible for breast and ovarian cancers in women and prostate cancer in men. They occur from the leaching of plastic bottles caused by hot temperatures[4]—for example, bottled water that is transported in hot trucks from hot warehouses or left in your car for too long. It's easy to see how premature aging, disease, and quality of life is affected just by drinking water from plastic bottles and containers!

Should our bodies become toxic for any length of time, the end result will be hormonal imbalances. That is why a healthy lifestyle plays a huge role in hormone balance and your overall state of well-being.

Q5: What healthy lifestyle practices are for restoring hormone balance?

A: 1) Food. As we age, our nutritional demands increase. To meet those demands properly, we must establish a solid nutritional base through the food we eat—our diet. We're not talking about dieting here but ensuring a solid base comes from compatible food for our blood type. In my experience, making food selections based on your blood type is most accurate.

2) Stem Cell Activation/Technology. Because of disruptive technologies like adult stem cell activators, we now can rejuvenate, repair, and restore the stem cells of the glands, organs, and in the case of hormones, the endocrine system. The major endocrine glands include the pineal gland, pituitary gland, pancreas, ovaries, testes, thyroid gland, parathyroid gland, and adrenal glands. Your endocrine system basically secretes hormones to meet your hormonal demands. As you age, this secretion process slows down and consequently you become hormone deficient and experience aging symptoms.

(See section 2 for information on the adult stem cell activator ENDO for men and women.) ENDO is the targeted activator for the stem cells in the endocrine system. The stem cell activation enhances normal gland and organ function. As organ function improves, hormone supply and secretions become readily available. Then our endocrine system is able to meet the body's hormone demands.

3) Nutritional Supplements. It's difficult, if not impossible, to meet all of our nutritional needs with food. That's why I recommend nutritional supplementation. There are many supplements that can be listed, but I would rather make it simple and concise. (Be sure to check with your doctor before taking any supplements.)

Taking supplements like melatonin is good for inducing deeper, more recuperative, more restful sleeping patterns. This then translates to a more energetic next day, including increased mental sharpness, more excitement, a desire to go out and do things, and just living more vibrantly.

Powerful antiaging supplements DHEA and HGH help raise the

natural hormonal levels in the body to enhance energy levels, restore sexual performance, and bolster the immune system.

Antioxidants are nutrient substances that function as scavengers, neutralizing free radical molecules. They oppose oxidation and inhibit reactions promoted by oxidation. Some antioxidants that can be taken as dietary supplements are vitamin A, vitamin E, selenium, beta-carotene, coenzyme Q10, zinc, and green tea.

Super antioxidants that range from twenty to fifty times the potency of vitamins C and E are called *proanthocyanidins*. They are generally extracted from grapeseed and are very potent yet nontoxic.

All antioxidants contribute to strengthening the heart muscles, cleaning the arteries, lowering cholesterol, fighting cancer, and reducing swelling from arthritic pain.

For men, the prostate needs certain nutrients to keep it healthy, functioning properly, and resilient well into their later years. A healthy prostate will enhance sexual performance and help offset potential prostate cancer.

4) Regular Exercise. Without sounding redundant, exercise must be a part of one's lifestyle. Exercise is a natural dynamic necessary for preventative and recuperative measures for safeguarding optimal health. The opposite, which is a sedentary lifestyle, is plagued with premature illnesses and diseases such as diabetes, elevated blood pressure and cholesterol, weak immune system, poor cardiovascular health, poor circulation, lack of joint support, chronic pain, gastrointestinal problems, low or no libido or sex life, and much more. Exercise will boost your energy levels and mental acuteness, stimulate the circulatory system, reduce cholesterol, strengthen weak and sore joints, boost the immune system, and build muscle tissue for fat burning and body stability.

Healthy living benefits from exercise:

- Functional ability grows. Strength training makes everyday tasks easier and helps people keep their independence.

- Arthritic-like pain and disability lessens. Strength training strengthens joints and increases joint lubrication and stability.

- Bones become stronger. Strength training fights osteoporosis by increasing bone mineral density. The increased strength of bones, muscles, and connective tissue causes a decrease in the risk of injury.

- The mind becomes healthier. Strength training improves mental alertness and self-worth, which fights depression—a condition that has become more and more common among our seniors.

- Insulin sensitivity improves. Strength training improves insulin sensitivity and glucose regulation, which stabilizes blood sugar. This contributes to a steady energy level.

- A greater quality of life and extended functional independence is experienced. As a rule, people who maintain their physical strength can perform everyday activities and tasks much easier and well past their retirement days.

Regular exercise, eating foods compatible with your blood type, and dietary supplementation are the keys for healthy longevity. Hormonal control and balance are also necessary for both men and women to experience a good quality of life.

As you can see, the role of hormones is so huge that they should be treated as the base for supporting a healthy body both now and into our future years. I hope you can see that the aging process and its related health issues, diseases, and symptoms are linked to hormonal levels, not our age. With that in mind you are better equipped to address the proper areas in your body to live a long, healthy, vibrant, and pain-free life.

CHAPTER 11

THE DETOX

ESTABLISHING A NUTRITIONAL base, like I mentioned earlier in chapter 8, is very crucial to your overall health. If you are supplying your body with nutrients from the proper food sources for cellular sustainability, it only stands to reason that the food sources be the most biochemically compatible. This will ensure proper uptake and assimilation of the nutrients from the food.

Your body's nourishment takes place at the cellular level via the bloodstream. All nutrients, oxygen, and other essential elements are likewise carried to the multitrillion cellular networks for conversion.

Once your nutritional base is in place, you can start targeting areas of concern, such as diseases. All diseases are caused by a combination of parasites, environmental toxins, bad bacteria, viruses, toxic foods, stress, and even mineral deficiencies. When the toxic load is too much, you have imbalance, which causes, for lack of a better word, disease.

The first line of defense when addressing disease is to detox the body. By making food selections for your blood type, you go through natural detoxification. By avoiding foods that are incompatible with your blood type, you are removing the foods that are toxic for your body chemistry. That natural detoxification reduces painful joints, lowers cholesterol, increases energy, and reduces fat cell size. As you make food selections for your blood type, the toxins that are built up in the fat cells (from the incompatible foods eaten prior) will dissipate and you lose excess weight.

To protect your body from becoming toxic or developing auto-intoxication and a litany of poor health conditions, the final process of the alimentary canal (also called digestive tract), expelling solid wastes, must be addressed.

Without the proper and regular elimination of solid wastes, your colon will become a stagnant cesspool of built-up mucus and hardened fecal matter, which is a breeding bed for parasitic infestation—the perfect time bomb for imploding your health.

COLON HEALTH: DETOXIFICATION

I am a firm proponent that disease starts in the colon. When the colon is functioning properly, the result will be good health, but when dysfunctional, one will experience poor health. To establish a healthy lifestyle, starting with the colon is a brilliant strategy. Therefore, as I myself, my wife, and perhaps thousands of my clients do, I recommend you do a colon cleanse as the first step toward improving your health.

The first line of defense when addressing disease is to detox the body.

Before you can ever expect an organ, gland, or bodily system to heal and be restored to natural function, you must detoxify your body—eliminate toxins. As you start out making healthy lifestyle changes to minimize or eliminate illnesses or any poor health condition, you must cleanse your colon. I cannot express this fact strongly enough. The healing process cannot take place if your body is toxic.

A dysfunctional colon plays a major role in most degenerative diseases. A dysfunctional colon involves a slow *transit time*, which is the time it takes to eliminate the solid waste from the food that has been ingested. This slowing of the transit time in most cases is caused by *constipation*. If you do not have two or three bowel movements per day, you are considered clinically constipated—at least in my world of naturopathy; not so much by medical community standards.

I have had personal conversations with an orthopedic surgeon specializing in pain management who disagrees with my definition of constipation. He stated he was not all that concerned about his patients being constipated until they surpassed seven days—a whole week! Really? Let's see how that translates in relation to your overall health.

TRANSIT TIME

The transit time of a healthy colon is approximately sixteen to twenty-four hours. When the transit time is slowed down due to constipation (average American adult transit time is estimated to be ninety-six hours), a buildup of toxins from impacted fecal matter begins. Mucus and fecal matter that become impacted into the porous walls of the colon not only cause digestive inflammatory pain and discomfort, but they also lead to more serious conditions such as diverticulitis, IBS, diverticulosis, polyps, and worse, cancer of the colon.

The longer toxins remain in the colon, the greater the chances for disease to develop and the more time they have to catch a ride in the bloodstream (a condition called leaky gut or leaky colon). Once in the bloodstream this toxic waste circulates throughout your body, polluting it and breaking down your quality of health. This putrefied condition overloads the liver, causing it to take on more of a workload, and will potentially weaken it.

The health of your colon is also directly related to the health of your blood. Since life is in the blood, it would behoove everyone to detox.

Causes of Constipation

There are several factors that cause constipation:

- a lack of exercise
- dehydration; not drinking enough water
- eating refined flour and refined sugar products, fried foods, and deli food
- lack of dietary fiber
- taking medications
- stress

Constipation can be corrected by making healthy lifestyle changes.

PARASITES AND YOUR HEALTH

Just the thought of having parasites living within your colon is about the most disgusting thing imaginable. Constipation makes your colon a breeding bed for parasitic infestation. Yet people go day in and day out without a bowel movement, never realizing the presence of their rent-free tenants.

And if all this is not enough to make you vomit, listen to this. Parasites have an approximate thirty-six-hour window for incubation. If your colon is healthy and functioning properly, you should have regular bowel movements (within that twenty-four-hour transit time) after ingesting that last meal and not have to deal with the next health concern: overgrowth of parasites.

Before you can ever expect an organ, gland, or bodily system to heal and be restored to natural function, you must detoxify your body... The healing process cannot take place if your body is toxic.

But on the other hand, if your colon is not functioning properly, then there is a good chance you are like most adults who have an average transit time of ninety-six hours. Now this sickening dilemma lends itself to plenty of time for those scurvy little maggot-like parasites to incubate and grow or colonize.

Once these parasites work their way into your colon, they do a couple of things: first, they eat what you ate; and second, they excrete their feces into your body via your bloodstream while building their breeding colonies. These parasites range from single-cell amoebae to four-inch worms, spreading their toxic refuse throughout your body, which eventually weakens and interrupts your health.

Parasitic infestation contributes to a litany of health-related problems like liver dysfunction, degenerative diseases, headaches, achy joints, weakness, weak immune system, skin ailments, poor skin tone, bad breath, and many more. Knowing this information about the colon only begs the question, why would I ever suggest to my patients that being constipated up to seven days is not anything to be concerned with, like the orthopedic doctor?

TESTIMONIAL

October 15, 2012

I have personally been using this product (INNER OUT colon cleansing system) since 2002! I saw Dr. Joseph Christiano on Daystar talking about feeling sluggish, skin problems, indigestion, etc., and the body's need for a colon cleanse. He named a lot of reasons why we all need to cleanse, but he mentioned the necessity of cleansing if one has been on a lot of medication such as antibiotics.

Well, my twenty-five-year-old son had been in a car wreck, went into a coma, [and] had half of his skull removed and put in the freezer. For three months, he was given several strong medications. When they put his skull back on, he was given intravenously the strongest antibiotics available and multiple kinds so his body wouldn't reject his skull. Now this is the reason I became so sold on this unique colon cleanse that scrubs your colon walls.

You see, almost two years after my son's wreck, his complexion was so bad. It was hard for him to accept because he never had acne as a teen and was always complimented on his beautiful face. After watching the show, I decided to place an order for myself and my son. I did mine first and honestly felt twenty years younger! Then my son, Joshua, did it.

I was thinking about all the prescriptions he had been on for so long, but had completely forgot about the feeding tube he had for nine months. The day his feeding tube was placed, they ran a bag of some turquoise radioactive dye through his system to ensure that it was placed correctly.

I was in absolute shock and awe as the colon cleanse scrubbed all nine feet of his colon. For three days, he produced nine feet of turquoise you know what! IMMEDIATELY I remembered that radioactive dye hanging from the pole next to his bed. I also remembered that at the nursing home when they would disconnect a feeding bag from his tube that it would drip on the floor. If it would dry without being wiped up, then it would take a razor blade, not a paring knife to get it removed. It was like hard rubber when it dried. Joshua's colon was lined with this stuff for two years!

This amazing product scrubbed it clean, like new. His complexion immediately cleared up and even better than that is his memory became so clear, no more short-term memory loss. He was back to normal and we became completely sold on this God-breathed product of Dr. Joseph Christiano and have many friends and family using it now. Thank you, Dr. Christiano!

—DEBRA H.

If you or someone you know are taking medications, please make colon cleansing and detoxifying a priority. Medications are a very real toxic culprit and cause multiple digestive problems to the colon.

DETOX AND YOUR HEALTH

Spring/Fall Cleaning

Ideally, a colon cleansing system that I believe is most thorough and effective is a two-week, three-phase system. (See the appendix for information on this program.) Instead of taking herbal laxatives or trying to manage a thirty-day cleanse, I find that a two-week system that works in phases is most complete and doable for anyone regardless of their schedule or health. Remember, consult your physician first if you have health conditions or are taking medications.

INNER OUT

Phase 1, or the Preparation Phase, lasts for seven days. During this phase, you will take an herbal complex supplement in capsule form both in the morning and in the evening. You do not have to change anything with regards to eating or taking medications and supplements. During the preparation phase, the colon is being prepared for the cleansing phase by removing built-up mucus from the colon walls. Parasites are also killed, and their dwelling places are eliminated.

Phase 2, or the Detoxifying and Cleansing Phase, lasts for four days. These four days you will go on a liquid-only juice fast. Avoiding solid foods is necessary if you want to remove all the impacted fecal matter, parasites, and mucus.

During this phase, you likewise take the capsules as directed and make four cleansing drinks with the cleansing powder (bentonite clay) in the juice of your choice. This phase really makes things start happening!

The bentonite clay has a dual action: it scrubs the porous walls of the colon and is a powerful absorption agent. The clay absorbs the mucoid and parasites that were destroyed in Phase 1.

Phase 3, or the Restoration Phase, is simply breaking the juice fast and returning to normal eating. This phase includes taking probiotics for replacing good bacteria in the gut. Now the colon is ready to eliminate properly the solid waste material that may have been stored in the colon for months and even years.

The results vary among everyone who goes through a colon cleanse, but your body will absorb nutrients from the foods you eat much more efficiently. You will experience more energy from the fruits and vegetables as the nutrients are better assimilated throughout the body, and you will have the mental satisfaction of knowing you just made a brilliant healthy lifestyle choice for the prevention of possible future damaging diseases and degenerative illness. There's nothing like a Spring and Fall Detox. (See INNER OUT colon cleansing system in the appendix.)

Healthy living is a process and lifelong endeavor. It has never been a short-term goal or ninety-day wonder. It has a positive impact in every area of your life. By including these key components I mentioned, you will experience all that I am saying as it becomes a natural part of your daily life.

CHAPTER 12

STRESS AND RELAXATION

S TRESS AND RELAXATION—NOW there's an example of polar opposites if I ever heard one. Though they should function together like hand and glove, the yin and the yang, unfortunately that is not the case for most people. Most often we tip the scales on the stress side.

STRESS

There is no doubt that you and I have too much stress in our lives. Most of the time we run around with our plates overflowing with an extraordinarily long list of things to do. To top that off, we need it all done yesterday. We are driven with deadlines and sales goals, or the daily routine of picking up and dropping off the kids. We learned to multitask when we were kids or we could never have kept up with the demands of the day. We unintentionally put ourselves under constant stress that ultimately is playing havoc on our health.

This topic always reminds me of when Lori and I got married in Jamaica. Having an all-inclusive wedding and honeymoon package for two weeks really taught us how to relax. Maybe it was the steel drum musicians playing the swaying Caribbean music, or the constant sound from the water falls that surrounded our resort that helped us learn to chill out. I remember talking to a Jamaican guy who made me realize I wasn't totally aware of how stressed we Americans are. This Jamaican attendant at our resort told me he noticed that when Americans came to the resort it took them several days to de-stress. He said, "Hey, mon, what's da hurry? You dudes are gonna die of heart attacks if you don't slow down."

AUTONOMIC NERVOUS SYSTEM

Allow me to show you where the real action is taking place when your stress and relaxation duo are out of balance—your autonomic nervous system (ANS). Your body's stress hormone levels are regulated by the ANS, which functions to regulate the body's unconscious actions. It has two parts to it: the sympathetic nervous system (SNS) and the parasympathetic nervous system (PNS). Let's start with the sympathetic nervous system since that is the system we use most of the time.

In response to a stressor, the sympathetic nervous system orchestrates what we call the fight-or-flight response. When activated, this system increases muscle blood flow and tension, dilates pupils, accelerates heart rate and respiration, and increases perspiration and arterial blood pressure. These symptoms can be felt every time you are in a stressful situation. This could happen just before you do a presentation, when you are involved in a confrontation with your spouse, or when you are following someone who is texting while driving.

Once the stressful event is over, the body should return to normal physiological function, making you and I feel more at ease. The problem is that we don't always calm down because we are constantly overstressed. Unless we make some changes, we will keep our sympathetic nervous system revving all the time and eventually be dealing with all sorts of health problems starting with adrenal fatigue, hypercortisolism, or Cushing's syndrome. Let me share a scenario with you. Imagine you are on an African safari and a lion appears in front of you. Naturally you are scared out of your mind, so you take off running—the fight-or-flight response. Hopefully you find protection, the chase ends, and your SNS can return to normal.

Now imagine yourself sitting in your chair at the office thinking about the never-ending cycle of deadlines, sales quotas, a coworker who takes credit for your ideas, the promotion or raise you didn't get, or whatever stresses you about your job. Maybe you're retired but your adult son or daughter is struggling with serious problems, or a financial setback is causing daily stress and anxiety in your life. Maybe you stay at home with your young children and you feel the stress of comparing yourself to other moms as you try to "do it all" and live up to false standards of perfection. Whatever it is, instead of being calm and relaxed, your sympathetic nervous system is running in high gear, like the lion is still chasing you and you haven't found a haven of protection, so to speak, where you can calm down. What next?

The other part of the autonomic nervous system is the parasympathetic nervous system. This is the part of the involuntary nervous system that serves to slow the heart rate, increase intestinal and glandular activity, and relax the sphincter muscles. When this part is in play, it reverses those symptoms/responses that happen when you and I are being chased by the lion. This is the system that kicks in once the other system (SNS) is shut off so we can relax.

RELAXATION

Perhaps you have seen what actors or musicians do just before they perform—they take a deep breath or two. This is referred to as a diaphragmatic breathing or belly breathing exercise. While operating from the sympathetic nervous system, we tend to take short, shallow breaths. In fact, when we are stressed, we are forced to breathe that way.

There is a nerve that controls our parasympathetic nervous system or our relaxation response. It is called the *vagus* nerve. This nerve releases the neurotransmitter acetylcholine, which is responsible for calming and relaxing the body. It sends electrical messages of peace and relaxation throughout the body via stimulation of the parasympathetic nervous system (PNS).

One simple exercise to stimulate the vagus nerve to release acetylcholine is belly or diaphragmatic breathing. This form of exercise for relaxation is simple to do, can be done anywhere at any time, and is extremely helpful. Here is what you need to do.

To practice proper diaphragmatic breathing, it is best to lie down on the couch, bed, or floor. Place a book on your stomach and take a deep breath. If you are performing this breathing exercise properly, the book will rise and lower throughout the exercise.

As you inhale you are directing the air through your belly, allowing the four cavities of your lungs to fill with air. You will notice your belly swell out and the book will rise and lower as you exhale.

Simply inhale (pushing your belly out) through your mouth, allowing as much air to fill your lungs as possible, and then exhale very slowly through your tightly closed lips. Repeat this exercise several times until you start feeling less stressed—it really does work! Of course, you don't have to lie down to do this exercise once you know how to do it.

When it comes to relaxation, you need to get creative. You must take a proactive approach or you will stay overstressed and eventually become sick.

Stress is all too common among most people, but relaxation is not. Therefore, my suggestion is to determine ways to cut back on your stressful conditions when possible. For each stressful situation, there is a counterpunch for stress reduction. Maybe your career choice is far too stressful and it is ruining the happiness and satisfaction you thought your career would deliver. Then it might be time to change careers, or at least change the company you work for within that career.

And for those things you can't change, there are ways to manage your stress. Maybe a relationship is getting too stressful day in and day out. You might want to consider professional counseling if it is a spouse or parent/child relationship. If it is a friend or acquaintance, consider putting healthy limits or boundaries on the relationship to reduce your stress.

If you're stressed because you're always late—whether it's picking up your kids from school, paying the electric bill, showing up for an appointment or meeting, or getting to the airport on time—try creating a daily schedule that builds more margin (more time) for you to get these things done instead of waiting until the last minute or being unrealistic about how much time it really takes.

And be sure to take time out to find something to be thankful for each and every day. The mental, emotional, and spiritual benefits of gratitude cannot be underestimated, and this in turn helps reduce your body's stress response.

My point is, stress reduction is extremely important because it affects your entire life.

When it comes to relaxation, you need to get creative. You must take a proactive approach or you will stay overstressed and eventually become sick. When Lori and I first married, one of the topics we discussed was getting away. I always felt it important for us to get away for some "we time" so we could enjoy each other and get away from the hustle and bustle of life. I had been insistent from the beginning that we would not wait until we retire to travel or enjoy life.

We make it a point to get away as often as we can, whether it is a short weekend at the beach or a seven-day cruise or anything in between. The result has been a good balance between stress and relaxation.

As you make healthy lifestyle changes, keep a balance between stress and relaxation on the top of the list. That balancing act will play a huge role in your overall healthy living journey.

THE FINAL WORD

I N THIS CONCLUSION, I would like to review what I've written about in this book and bring everything into perspective. As you and I look forward to living a healthy, pain- and disease-free, vibrant life, we must become smart patients, excellent caretakers of our health, wise with our choice of treatment options, and steeped in a preventative and proactive mentality that keeps us best prepared for what the future brings.

As you go beneath the surface of your visible outward appearance and physique, you know there is a cellular network of multiple trillions of cells that do amazingly incredible things to keep you healthy and functioning normally. When this network of cells is communicating and signaling to one another properly—repairing and fixing damaged cells to keep this human machinery in tip-top running order—all is well!

But truth be told, we understand that through environmental toxins, physical trauma, sickness, disease, stress, and the aging process, our cells get damaged, are less effective, and if unattended will ultimately put our healthy tip-top physiology into a downward tailspin.

There is no doubt in my mind that science and medicine have made leaps and bounds in technological advancements, treatments, and therapies over the decades. Conventional medicine is like the bunny in the battery commercials that keeps on going. However, it has its limitations and is overdue for much-needed improvements in the handling of patients' health conditions.

Being dosed with toxic medications to "heal" a physiological problem has never worked, yet that is a common medical practice. Being held hostage to myriad prescriptions to treat symptoms rather than the root cause of the problem has been a financially profitable endeavor for the practitioner and "Big Pharma," but the patient has become the victim of additional multiple health problems associated with the medications prescribed.

My goal in writing this book was to provide you with information that would shift your mind-set and inspire you to become a smart patient. If I've succeeded, I hope the idea of trusting your health to conventional medicine as your only treatment option now leaves much to be desired.

POSITIVE DISRUPTIONS

Freedom can be a good thing, especially the freedom to choose healthy options for our lives. We live in a time when having "options" is a buzzword for making a choice. Whether at a buffet on a cruise ship, at the salon deciding which type of nail color, or choosing the color schemes for the rooms in your house, the options are endless!

But to take full advantage of this freedom, we need to wake up to all of the options that are truly available to us. It's time to think outside the box that limits you to conventional medical treatments and discover there are many other effective treatment options available to you. Become a smart patient and you will naturally seek newer and more advanced options for your medical care and conditions.

> *Today the smart patient has a huge list of options before them to choose from when dealing with musculoskeletal problems and degenerative illnesses.*

Today you and I are living in very exciting times. We are witnessing revolutionary changes in the financial world as well as in the fields of medicine and science. Look at the transformation of our way of making payments. We have gone from bartering mined gold for goods, to paper and coin money to buy and sell, to digital money like debit cards and PayPal. Now cryptocurrency is very quickly becoming the new norm by which one will buy and sell. This is referred to as "disruptive technology."

In science and medicine, the conventional approach to treating patients is also being replaced by a new norm—stem cell therapies, treatments, and activators. Today the smart patient has a huge list of options before them to choose from when dealing with musculoskeletal problems and degenerative illnesses. Prior to these disruptive treatments, we were limited in what options were available to us, such as the litany of medications, surgical procedures, and health-damaging chemical therapies.

Until now it sounded like science fiction to imagine a time when medical physicians could take their patients' own God-given genetic material—with zero complications, rejections, or the need for toxic medications or other foreign material—and use it for healing, repairing, and bringing pain relief to those patients. But the truth is, *that time has arrived*. I am personally taking advantage of the new norms for the betterment of my current and future health, as are many men and women from all walks of life throughout the world.

Today, as alternative medicine such as naturopathy advances in its field of natural remedies, technologies, and protocols, you and I can treat ourselves using natural substances enhanced by cutting-edge technologies like nanotechnology. Over time, as our human bodies start to degenerate and deteriorate, our own natural repair crews—our adult stem cells—start losing their ability to keep our cells operating properly. Consequently, we start to live with nagging illnesses, chronic discomfort or pain, and loss of genuine optimum health.

To have access to these technologies and natural substances is the choice of the smart patient. The new norm for treating our own health conditions makes being a faithful caretaker of our health much more effective.

The typical cost of medical treatments in the past can now be greatly reduced and possibly eliminated by circumventing unaffordable cash outlays, additional co-pays, doctor visits, or medications. This is what the twenty-first-century smart patient is looking for when it comes to managing their health and improving their quality of life.

You and I cannot accept yesterday's standards or measurements to determine our health and that of our children and grandchildren for the future. New standards of practice and treatment are here and available like never before in the history of medicine and health care. But even with all of these magnificent cutting-edge technologies, treatments, and therapies, you and I must not depend solely on them. It is our personal obligation to be faithful caretakers of our health. As you know very well, if you don't do it—no one will!

THE JOURNEY

The intelligent patient today will search for a competent orthopedic physician or primary physician who thinks outside the box and is up on the latest technologies and treatments should their health take a turn for the worse. Or they can opt to visit a stem cell physician/specialist should they be in an auto accident, become injured, develop a degenerative disease, or be given the prognosis that a knee replacement surgery is needed. Now this smart patient, though having to be *reactive*, will have better options for restoration and healing at their disposal.

This is all well and good, but what about *proactive* responsibilities with your health? The goal in your healthy living journey is not seeing how much pain you can endure, but rather eliminating all the pain you can so you can truly enjoy your life. That should be your motivation for incorporating healthy lifestyle practices. As your physiology improves on the journey, your need to see a stem cell physician, orthopedic physician, or any physician can be greatly minimized. In a nutshell, it's like the old adage—an apple a day keeps the doctor away.

The responsibility lies on each of our shoulders as to whether we want a healthy life or not. It won't come without effort, so the amount of value we place on our quality of life should dictate how much effort we will invest in this journey. Let's face it, we all can find the time to do what we ought to do if we put a high enough priority on it.

When a person finds balance in their life, they have found a wonderful thing. The synergy that comes when you are in tune with your body is beyond priceless. This instinctive ability to know what works and doesn't work for your body is more than half the battle. That is why developing a positive mental attitude—the mental capacity that is more powerful than most realize—really sets the journey in motion.

Being mentally rather than emotionally driven, you are ready to take on the new changes. Ideally, you must start with a nutritional base that is both doable and adaptable, two critical components for long-term survival. When food types align with your body chemistry, there is a genetic response that naturally puts the body into *homeostasis* (balance). This nutritional base along with nutritional supplements, supplies the body with the best means for assimilation of the nutrients from the food types they consume. The body also naturally detoxifies and induces the perpetuity of an energetic, vibrant, pain- and disease-free life. (See my book *Bloodtypes, Bodytypes, and You* in the appendix.)

When a person finds balance in their life,
they have found a wonderful thing.

Genetically we were not designed or created to be sedentary. That is why sedentariness is a precursor to health problems. But the good news is that the human body will adapt to stimulus, so any form of regular physical activity, whether it is a walking program, participating in sports, or hitting the gym, can counteract the downside of living a sedentary life.

It is not always a matter of laziness or being accustomed to a life of physical inactivity. Many people have fallen prey to advancements in technology in such a way that it has created a litany of health problems. Just to combat the hours of sedentariness at the workplace, you are almost forced to work out or do something physical—it is all about creating and sustaining a balance! In light of the recent research that reveals how sitting is as bad for your health as smoking, it would behoove you to get and stay physically active.

Don't forget how important your hormones are to your body's ability to repair itself, to protect you by slowing down the aging process, and to give you the benefits of youthful pleasures. Balancing your hormones is part of living a healthy life.

Because you are constantly exposed to environmental toxins and pollutants, infectious diseases, transmitted diseases, food additives, chemicals, and heavy metals, your body's ability to utilize the nutrients from your foods and supplements diminishes. Over time your body becomes toxic, which directly causes a premature decline in your immune system, induces autoimmune diseases, and interferes with or even prevents your body's ability to heal. Factoring in times throughout every year to detox your body is as important to your healthy living journey as avoiding secondhand smoke. Both will kill you eventually and most likely prematurely.

Lastly, don't underestimate the need to relax, destress, and let your body unwind. Do what you can to eliminate or manage stress, and take time out to relax and enjoy life as often as you can. Your health depends on it!

THE TIME IS NOW!

Unfortunately, it usually takes something traumatic to get a person's attention when it comes to change. Change is difficult for many people because it takes you out of your comfort zone. Most people are creatures of habit, so who wants to change?

But remember, you have been given life freely. Your body is so marvelously designed and fashioned that it can endure abuse for years and years without much indication. Yet at some point, it will start to break down. At some point down the road that ugly face of ill health will stop your life right in its tracks and tell you something you never want to hear—now you are mine!

Now is the time to do something disruptive about your health. Treat your health with a new approach. Don't wait until it's too late or you are forced to do something about it. Embrace your life, your new health options, and everything that matters to you. Your life is a gift that is meant to be enjoyed—develop a healthy life so you can do just that! Always remember, the journey it takes to reach your goals is designed to bring fulfillment and reward to you along the way, and throughout the process you will be watched by others who will be influenced by your example.

So, with every healthy step you take, keep in mind—you are an *inspiration in transition!*

PRODUCTS

W<small>E ALL KNOW</small> that supplementing our diet with additional nutrients helps fortify our body, making it more resilient, energetic, and vibrant. So, please take advantage of my nutritional products and services at www.bodyredesigning.com.

Listed below are just a few supplements/services related to this book topic.

INNER OUT COLON CLEANSING SYSTEM

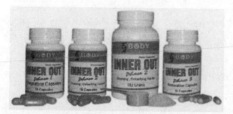

The Inner Out Colon Cleansing system is a 14-day, 2-week program designed to generate a progressive cleansing effect on your body in just 14 days. There are three important phases:

Phase 1: Preparation Phase—Prepares the colon. Helps kill off parasites, remove mucus from the colon walls, and may enhance bowel movement.

Phase 2: The Cleansing Phase—The primary colon cleansing and detoxifying effectiveness revolves around the ingredients found in the Phase 2 Cleansing and Detoxifying Powder. These ingredients team together with other nutrients in the capsules to perform a proper colon cleansing and detoxifying process. The claylike substance has a scrubbing action and a 100:1 absorption power that cleans the wall of the colon and removes toxic buildup and parasites.

Phase 3: The Restoration Phase—Return to eating solids. Take the herbal formula capsules containing probiotics for replenishing good bacteria into your colon.

Cleansing is a great asset in the maintenance of optimum health. Dr. Joe recommends a colon cleanse every six months for optimum health.

For more information, visit www.bodyredesigning.com or call 1-800-259-2639.

BLOODTYPES, BODYTYPES, AND YOU

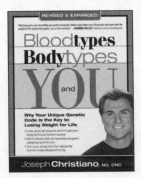

This best seller has been revised and expanded. You will learn how and why to eat foods designed specifically for your blood type—which foods you should eat and which you should avoid for your blood type. Enjoy fourteen varieties of breakfast, lunch, and dinner, plus desserts, snacks, hundreds of recipes, and *more!*

Dr. Joe's book explains how your blood type is pivotal in food selection for improving body composition that determines your ability to lose weight and keep it off for life. By making food selections for your blood type, you will discover how your body can eliminate painful joint inflammation, painful digestive disorders, gas, bloating, constipation, IBS, and sleepless nights.

Also improve your illness profile, lower cholesterol and blood pressure levels, reduce arthritic-like pain, and help stabilize your blood sugar!

"The most accurate and individualized way to eat that improves all areas of your life."—Dr. Joe

For more information, visit www.bodyredesigning.com or call 1-800-259-2639.

HOME BLOOD TYPING KIT

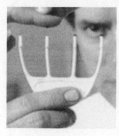

All the materials you need to take one blood type test is in this simple home blood typing kit. Within fifteen minutes you can know your blood type. Pretreated mixing card prevents misapplying or cross-contaminating anti-sera. Control panel on mixing card assures reliability. Just read instructions and follow directions for easy testing.

The home blood typing kit comes with: Eldoncard for ABO/Rh, mixing sticks, lancet, alcohol prep, and water pipette. Order one for each family member!

For more information, visit www.bodyredesigning.com or call 1-800-259-2639.

CONCENTRACE - LIQUID TRACE MINERALS

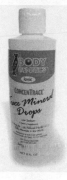

CONCENTRACE Liquid Minerals is a purified concentrated mineral source: a (desalinated) product providing mineral balance for more effective electric connections to nerve endings for alertness and body responses. Many arthritics with bone spurs have taken CONCENTRACE with successful results, dissolving abnormal mineral deposit spurs (bone spurs) and increasing energy and alertness. The dosage recommended on the product increases bowel action and eliminates the problem quickly. For more information, visit www.bodyredesigning.com or call 1-800-259-2639.

ADULT STEM CELL ACTIVATORS

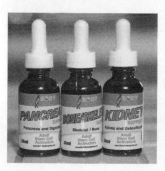

Adult Stem Cell Activators are designed to naturally repair and rejuvenate one's damaged or dormant adult stem cells. When our adult stem cells are healthy and functioning properly, we can experience less pain and discomfort, a new grip on our health, and a much greater quality of life! There are twenty-six targeted adult stem cell activators that are specifically designated for twenty-six different areas in the body, e.g., kidneys, pancreas, ligaments/tendons, liver, lungs, heart, nervous system, joints, weight loss, etc.

"It has been my personal and professional experience that these 'activators' provide the means to address the 'root cause' of one's disorder, disease and/or condition with efficacious results." —Dr. Joe

Everyone responds differently. Some experience immediate positive results while others may take longer. It is based on one's condition, be it chronic or acute, age, state of health, etc.

For more information call 1-800-259-2639 or visit www.body redesigning.com.

BASIC AND SPECIFIC NUTRITIONAL SUPPLEMENTS

1. **AM/PM MULTIVITAMINS**

2. **B-VITAMIN COMPLEX (for women)**

3. **PROST-EZE (for men)**

4. **COOLED OFF and TURMERIC 750mg (pain)**

5. **IMMUNE SUPPORT**

6. **HGH SUPPORT**

7. **WOMAN'S SUPPORT**

8. **TRIM (weight loss)**

9. **DIGESTIVE COMPLEX (digestive disorders)**

To order any of my products, please go to www.bodyredesigning.com or call 1-800-259-2639.

NEED A STEM CELL PHYSICIAN?

If you want to speak with a stem cell physician, please take advantage of my online **Virtual Directory for Stem Cell Physicians**. This website is designed to help you locate the nearest stem cell physician in your area. Simply visit http://stemcelldocs.net/ or call my office at 1-800-259-2639 and we will be glad assist you.

NOTES

EPIGRAPH

1. Mike Pence, "Pence Opposes Federal Funding of Destructive Embryonic Stem Cell Research," Vote Smart, January 10, 2007, https://votesmart.org/public-statement/233318/pence-opposes-federal-funding-of-destructive-embryonic-stem-cell-research#.WclhwciGPcs.

PREFACE: THE GAME CHANGER

1. Bob Pisani, "Bank Fees Have Been Growing Like Crazy," CNBC, July 21, 2017, https://www.cnbc.com/2017/07/21/the-crazy-growth-of-bank-fees.html.

CHAPTER 1: WHAT ARE STEM CELLS?

1. Ian Murnaghan, "History of Stem Cell Research," Explore Stem Cells, updated April 23, 2017, http://www.explorestemcells.co.uk/historystemcellresearch.html.

2. Murnaghan, "History of Stem Cell Research,"

3. Ian Murnaghan, "Stem Cell Research Around the World," Explore Stem Cells, May 14, 2017, http://www.explorestemcells.co.uk/StemCellResearchAroundWorld.html.

4. A. Manosroi et al., "In Vitro and In Vivo Skin Anti-Aging Evaluation of Gel Containing Niosomes Loaded with a Semi-Purified

Fraction Containing Gallic Acid from Terminalia Chebula Galls,"
Pharmaceutical Biology 49, no. 11 (November 2011): 1190–1203,
https://doi.org/10.3109/13880209.2011.576347.

5. J. I. Wolfstadt et al., "Current Concepts: The Role of Mesenchymal Stem Cells in the Management of Knee Osteoarthritis,"
Sports Health 7, no. 1 (January 2015): 38–44, https://doi.org/10.1177
/1941738114529727.

6. Phil Sneiderman, "Stem Cell Research: Joint Repair," Johns
Hopkins Medicine, accessed October 4, 2017, http://www.hopkins
medicine.org/stem_cell_research/coaxing_cells/joint_repair.html.

CHAPTER 2: ADULT STEM CELL THERAPY OPTIONS

1. Bradley Richard Hughes Jr., "Real-World Successes of Adult
Stem Cell Treatments," Life Issues Institute, December 1, 2004,
https://www.lifeissues.org/2004/12/real-world-successes-adult-stem
-cell-treaments.

CHAPTER 3: PRP—A DISRUPTIVE THERAPY

1. John J. Wilson, "Platelet-Rich Plasma Injection Procedure," Ver-
itas Health, January 7, 2014, https://www.arthritis-health.com
/treatment/injections/platelet-rich-plasma-injection-procedure; see
also Santos F. Martinez, "Practical Guidelines for Using PRP in the
Orthopaedic Office," American Academy of Orthopaedic Surgeons,
September 10, 2010, http://www.aaos.org/news/aaosnow/sep10
/clinical3.asp.

2. "Knee Osteoarthritis and Platelet Rich Plasma Therapy Injections," GetProlo.com, accessed October 4, 2017, http://www.getprolo
.com/knee-osteoarthritis-platelet-rich-plasma-therapy-injections/;
see also Wen-Li Dai et al., "Efficacy of Platelet-Rich Plasma in the
Treatment of Knee Osteoarthritis: A Meta-analysis of Randomized
Controlled Trials," *Arthroscopy* 33, no. 3 (March 2017): 659–70, http://
dx.doi.org/10.1016/j.arthro.2016.09.024.

3. "Knee Osteoarthritis and Platelet Rich Plasma Therapy Injections"; see also Longxiang Shen et al., "The Temporal Effect of
Platelet-Rich Plasma on Pain and Physical Function in the Treatment of Knee Osteoarthritis: Systematic Review and Meta-Analysis

of Randomized Controlled Trials," *Journal of Orthopaedic Surgery and Research* 12, no. 1 (January 23, 2017): 16, https://doi.org/10.1186 /s13018-017-0521-3.

4. "Knee Osteoarthritis and Platelet Rich Plasma Therapy Injections"; W. Kanchanatawan et al., "Short-Term Outcomes of Platelet-Rich Plasma Injection for Treatment of Osteoarthritis of the Knee," *Knee Surgery, Sports Traumatology, Arthroscopy* 24, no. 5 (May 2016): 1665–77, https://doi.org/10.1007/s00167-015-3784-4.

5. "Knee Osteoarthritis and Platelet Rich Plasma Therapy Injections"; Ryosuke Sakata and A. Hari Reddi, "Platelet-Rich Plasma Modulates Actions on Articular Cartilage Lubrication and Regeneration," *Tissue Engineering: Part B* 22, no. 5 (October 2016): 408–19, https://doi.org/10.1089/ten.TEB.2015.0534.

6. "Knee Osteoarthritis and Platelet Rich Plasma Therapy Injections"; Sakata and Reddi, "Platelet-Rich Plasma Modulates Actions on Articular Cartilage Lubrication and Regeneration."

7. "Knee Osteoarthritis and Platelet Rich Plasma Therapy Injections"; Sakata and Reddi, "Platelet-Rich Plasma Modulates Actions on Articular Cartilage Lubrication and Regeneration"; Ryosuke Sakata et al., "Stimulation of the Superficial Zone Protein and Lubrication in the Articular Cartilage by Human Platelet-Rich Plasma," *The American Journal of Sports Medicine* 43, no. 6 (June 2015): 1467–73, https://doi.org/10.1177/0363546515575023.

CHAPTER 5: THE SCIENCE BEHIND ADULT STEM CELL ACTIVATORS

1. For more information, visit http://www.protomed.org.

CHAPTER 10: ANTIAGING

1. Diana Gerstacker, "Sitting Is the New Smoking: Ways a Sedentary Lifestyle Is Killing You," *Huffington Post*, updated November 26, 2014, http://www.huffingtonpost.com/the-active-times/sitting-is-the -new-smokin_b_5890006.html.

2. Gerstacker, "Sitting Is the New Smoking"; Mary MacVean, "'Get Up!' or Lose Hours of Your Life Every Day, Scientist Says," *Los Angeles Times*, July 31, 2014, http://www.latimes.com/science /sciencenow/la-sci-sn-get-up-20140731-story.html.

3. Danielle Sedbrook, "2,4-D: The Most Dangerous Pesticide You've Never Heard Of," Natural Resources Defense Council, March 15, 2016, https://www.nrdc.org/stories/24-d-most-dangerous-pesticide-youve-never-heard.

4. Atonia M. Calafat et al., "Exposure of the U.S. Population to Bisphenol A and 4-Tertiary-Octylphenol: 2003–2004," *Environmental Health Perspectives* 116, no. 1 (January 2008): 39-44, https://www.ncbi.nlm.nih.gov/pmc/articles/PMC2199288/.

INDEX